A Year in the Life
of a "Dead" Woman

A Year in the Life of a "Dead" Woman

Living with Terminal Cancer

Lynnette Porter

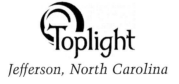

Toplight

Jefferson, North Carolina

ISBN (print) 978-1-4766-7896-2
ISBN (ebook) 978-1-4766-3865-2

Library of Congress Cataloguing Data are available

British Library cataloguing data are available

Front cover image © 2019 Shutterstock

Printed in the United States of America

Toplight is an imprint of McFarland & Company, Inc., Publishers

*Box 611, Jefferson, North Carolina 28640
www.toplightbooks.com*

Table of Contents

Acknowledgments

Thank you to the many family members, good friends, and helpful, gracious teachers, mentors, and colleagues who have made my life special and shaped me into the woman I became. I especially acknowledge and express my love and gratitude for these very special people:

my parents, Charles Raymond Porter and Doris James Porter

my beloved brother, Bartley Alan Porter

my paternal grandparents, Charles Greenlee Porter and Mary Pauline Porter

my maternal grandmother, Margaret Marie McIntire (but always Mom-ma Margie to me)

my sister-in-law, Nancy; my niece, Heather; my great-nephew, Levi; and my great-niece, Ava

my "sister"/cousin, Janet Davis

my dear friend for more than fifty years, Genie Fyffe

my "sister," travel companion, and conscience, Jennifer Wojton

my "sister" and trusted advisor, Joy Carney

my extended family who "adopted" me: Chris, Layla, and Thomas Wojton; Lynn Carney; Carlos, Nico, and Roman Arias

my former department chair, great friend and supporter, and generous artist, quilt maker, and baker, Donna Barbie

Preface

Death is helping me make meaning out of my life. It provides opportunities for me to revisit some of my favorite literary works, television series, and films that have long influenced my outlook on life. T. S. Eliot wrote one of my favorite lines in his poem "Little Gidding," and, just as I have co-opted these words as part of my personal philosophical framework (which is far different from Eliot's intended meaning), so have some of my favorite characters. In the early 2000s, the BBC television series *Torchwood* (2006–2011) entertained me with the adventures of immortal time traveler Captain Jack Harkness (John Barrowman), no stranger to death. Stuck on Earth for centuries, Jack has frequently suffered the loss of friends and lovers. The series was originally set in Cardiff, Wales, where Jack headed Torchwood, an organization that monitors extraterrestrial life forms on Earth and protects the planet from alien incursions. Despite the cheesy alien-centric plots of the first two seasons, *Torchwood*'s stories force Captain Jack and his audience to confront the finality of death for mortals. In the second season finale episode, "Exit Wounds," two members of Torchwood die in the line of duty, leaving Jack and his two remaining colleagues to carry on despite the heavy loss. When his grieving compatriots wonder how they will go on, Jack explains that this ending (of their friends' lives and Torchwood as they knew it) becomes the point "where we start from," and the three surviving Torchwood team members adhere to this philosophy. *Torchwood* appropriated a line from Eliot's poem to offer advice not only from one television character to others but to a larger audience—and I have since used that context to better understand the human capacity to survive or even thrive after catastrophic events.

In director Peter Jackson's 2001 film adaptation of J. R. R. Tolkien's *The Lord of the Rings: The Fellowship of the Ring*, the wizard Gandalf

(Ian McKellen) memorably advises hobbit Frodo Baggins (Elijah Wood), "All we have to decide is what to do with the time that is given us." Frodo needs to hear these words near the beginning of what becomes an increasingly harrowing journey to defeat Evil; I needed to replay the video of them late one night while binge-watching Jackson's film trilogy soon after my diagnosis.

Filled with gratitude that I have been given time to live with a greater awareness of my mortality, I have chosen to write this memoir with both Captain Jack's and Gandalf's advice to guide me. The following chapters describe how I am living the remainder of my life, from indulgent travel to practical business, from personal introspection to professional interactions with colleagues, students, or strangers. Of course, because this book includes discussions of my cancer diagnosis and prognosis, my insights into cancer treatments and the state of U.S. health care are a recurring theme, but this is neither an inspirational tome nor an indictment of the medical institution. Instead, it is my story and, at times, that of my brother, father, and grandparents, who preceded me in death by cancer. Based on my and my family's experiences as cancer patients, many preconceptions about living with a terminal diagnosis and preparing for death are discussed. These preconceptions often lead to expectations for and by those who have cancer; what to expect when you or a family member is expected to die from cancer is more than a theme within this memoir—it is one of my purposes in writing this book.

Finally, because I am a lifelong pop culture nerd and fan-scholar, this memoir includes numerous references, such as those at the beginning of this Preface, to television series, books, films, and music as well as to actors, directors, authors, and singers. Throughout my life, I have attended fan events or performances and enjoyed chatting—however briefly—with, in particular, authors and actors whose work I admire. Creative works continue to inspire me, and I value the influence of popular culture in my life. Not only have such influences helped form my philosophy and become enmeshed in my spirituality, but they also have established many of my and others' preconceptions about the nature of death and, specifically, an often-terminal illness like cancer. Although I have long been an analyst of popular culture, a role that requires me to look at works for what they are, not what I or others wish them to be, I confess that, in this memoir, I have "read into" songs, dialogue, poems, and prose what stands out as important to me and have explained the context of those examples within my life. In short, I find myself doing what I have always told my students not to do: take meaning out of context. Although I still hold myself to that standard as I continue to write academic works, I have given myself permission to be far more flexible in writing my memoir.

An important limitation for this memoir is the timeframe. Whereas most memoirs provide a chronological overview of the author's life, from birth or childhood through the present, my focus is primarily on my life since April 2016, when I was first diagnosed with cancer. The "year in the life of a 'dead' woman" provides an even more focused look at my post-terminal diagnosis life from January to December 2018. However, because this is a memoir, I often digress chronologically to provide a broader context for my expectations, philosophy, or actions based on a lifetime of experiences.

Slightly more than the first half of the book (chapters 1 through 6) describes actions and activities—mine and others'—more than my philosophy of life or spiritual musings. The organizational shift from "activity" to "philosophy" (chapters 7 through 11) indicates my gradual real-life shift from an active, "normal"-appearing life to a more sedentary, introspective lifestyle in which I focus on my memories and analyses of aspects of life and death. Throughout the book, I refer to my mental separation of my body and my mind, although I know that the two are linked. However, this sense of physical/mental division since my cancer diagnosis has resulted in a revision and re-awareness of my self-identity, both physical and psychological/emotional. If this book is going to be all about me, I want to make sure I look critically at my life from both outside and inside, from my awareness of my body as well as my mind.

No "dead" woman is an island, even if she tries to retreat to Hawaii to escape her prognosis. The people closest to me, who should be credited for guiding and supporting me especially throughout my cancer journey, are identified by name. In a few instances, I shamelessly name-drop people famous at least within my fandoms and often to the general public. At other times, I refer to people only by occupation, such as "ophthalmologist," "oncologist," or "dentist." Those who fall in a "middle" category between close friends/family and famous people I do not know or may have briefly encountered are described in intentionally vague terms. I do not know how they would feel to be identified by name, but, if they read this memoir, they will know who they are. My lack of identification in no way reflects their professionalism, and, in fact, I am especially grateful to these people for their candor and humor.

Finally, because I often jump around chronologically as I discuss my experiences by theme, the following brief summary of my life between February 1957 and April 2016 should provide the necessary background to understand not only the context but specific geographical, pop culture, or familial references.

I was born in Evansville, Indiana, at 6:13 p.m. on Wednesday, February 27, 1957. I always appreciated knowing the exact place and time because, like my mother, Doris James (Jimmie) Goodman Porter, I enjoyed constructing and interpreting astrological charts. Mom and Dad, Charles Raymond (Ray) Porter, named their firstborn Lynnette Raye, although the local newspaper incorrectly listed the birth name as Lynnette Faye. Ironically, my first name was spelled correctly in the birth announcement; since then, many people have insisted on spelling it with only one n, to my frequent annoyance. Perhaps also ironically, Mom chose my name because she liked it in a story from a high school literature class: "Gareth and Lynette." Yes, this Lynette's name is correctly spelled, but, in the textbook Mom read, the name was published as "Lynnette," a spelling my mother preferred.

Despite some versions of the tale portraying Lynette as, at least, haughty and occasionally kind of a bitch, she often is portrayed as a magical being whose perseverance leads to her sister being freed from oppression by some less-than-chivalrous knights. I attribute my later love of Arthurian literature to my connection with Lynette. "Gareth and Lynette" also made my first kiss, Gary, even more attractive to my romantic heart because, I hoped, we might live a modernized fairy tale of "Gary and Lynette." When I later interviewed *Torchwood* actor Gareth David-Lloyd in Cardiff and hosted him in one of my university science fiction-themed Honors courses in Daytona Beach, I could not help but wistfully (perhaps a bit wishfully, too) connect my fondness for Gareth with my lifelong connection to "Gareth and Lynette."

However, my oldest cousin, Lynn Fortune, thinks that I may have been named for him, and, indeed, that's a possibility. Mom was always fond of Lynn. When he planned to marry Laurel McAlister in faraway

Massachusetts, Mom took six-year-old me with her when she accompanied her older sister and Lynn's mother, Helen, and my slightly older cousin Bonnie on the train ride to Boston. Not only did I love riding the train, but I adored the home of Laurel's parents on a rocky beach in—no kidding—Lynn, Massachusetts. I tasted lobster and a Shirley Temple for the first time. During the daylight hours free of wedding preparations, Bonnie and I were taken to places like Boston's Public Garden, where I was fascinated by the swan boats and a family friend let us each pick out a Kewpee doll from a lakeside vendor. At the McAlisters' oceanside home, I gingerly made my way down the rocky path to stick my toes in the water, finally giving up to search for little pieces of driftwood among the rocks. Despite trying to be very good and quiet, I caused a problem here or there. At the wedding reception, when everyone was encouraged to lift a glass of champagne to toast the newlyweds, Mom was too busy getting Bonnie and me to put down our glasses to enjoy the toast herself. (I liked the bubbles on my tongue. Like Laurel, who was shocked that her mother chose traditional Scottish fruitcake for the wedding cake, I didn't like the cake.) The multiple positive associations between Lynnette and the Lynns of the Massachusetts wedding were a good omen for my future, and the strongest memories associated with that trip—cross-country travel, beaches, lobster, and champagne—previewed what would be important to me later in life. To my mom's regret, my memories of the wedding itself are dim and possibly should have hinted that matrimonial institutions would not become a top priority for me.

Although Lynnette is intertwined with family and literary history, my middle name also has an interesting origin beyond my mom's appreciation of it. I was named for my dad, just as Mom was named for her father, James. Dad went by Ray, a short form of his middle name; James went by Jim. Mom "feminized" Ray by adding an e to the end. She also told me that I was her little ray of sunshine, which gave her a second reason to name me Raye. I think I ended up with the better name in honoring my father; Mom's middle name was James, and she was forever known as Jimmie.

As might be obvious from even this story of my naming, I was a much-wanted and -loved child, as was my brother, Bartley Alan, who arrived a little more than three years later. Bart and I were close; we played together and shared confidences. He was the kind of little brother who would appease my interest in playing schoolteacher by playing my student, even during summer vacations away from the classroom. He sat under the tree in our backyard on Bellemeade Avenue, going through the lesson I wrote on Mom's battered blackboard balanced on a tripod. A few years later, we created newspapers or comic books together, just for fun. Our favorite way of capturing our storytelling back then (when I was about 10 and Bart was seven) was to use my blue reel-to-reel tape recorder. Long after the recorder broke and technology speeded ahead, I carried those tapes with me as I moved from house to house, child to teen to adult; they became a tangible reminder of our earliest story-telling. As we grew older, Bart teased but protected me; he acted more like the older sibling. We always kept up with each other's life. Through-out our adulthood we frequently visited, emailed, or talked on the phone, no matter if we lived in the same city or hundreds of miles apart.

Bart and I shared a love of pop culture. We watched television together for hours each night when we were kids. We went to movies together as teens and young adults. He indulged my love of *Butch Cassidy and the Sundance Kid* (1969)—and Paul Newman, Robert Redford, and Katharine Ross—by taking me to see the movie three consecutive nights when it returned for a week's engagement at a local art house. He introduced me to *Star Wars* (1977) and made sure we watched the next two installments together on the day they came out. Bart saved movies on his VCR or DVR to watch with me when I visited him after he married. Many a weekend we shared the wee hours of the morning with Fritz the Night Owl or the *MST3K* crew.

Bart and I also were close because we were writers. Before he died (too early, in 2015, at 55), Bart told me that he wanted to be remembered as a writer, a fact I reiterated when I eulogized him. Bart became a journalist, a corporate communication specialist, and a fiction writer; I became a technical writer and editor, a teacher of writing, and the author or co-author of more than 20 non-fiction textbooks or pop culture studies. Always we shared our research and current projects with each other.

My childhood was happy and typical for a middle-class family in southern Indiana. I was a good student, especially at Hebron Elementary School and Harrison High School. I liked school—and having summers off—which likely formed the foundation for my future career as a technical writing consultant setting her own schedule and especially as a university professor on a nine-month-a-year contract. Shortly after my 1975 high school graduation, Dad took a promotion, and he, Mom, and Bart moved to Lima, Ohio. I remained in our hometown and became a student for one year at Indiana State University–Evansville; the final two of my three-year undergraduate career as a history major and radio/television/film minor were spent at Ball State University in Muncie. There I fell in love with the study of popular culture and was influenced by a classroom meeting with director Frank Capra. His knowledge of films and willingness to talk to students just beginning to learn about the history of film made me aware that at least part of my career could involve talking or writing about movies.

Before I returned to academia and writing, however, I bounced around Northwestern Ohio radio stations as an announcer and a deejay. Weird hours and low pay helped me to rethink what I really wanted to do with my life (which, it turned out, was writing) and to plan a way that I could make enough money that I could afford the time to write. I was employed briefly as a librarian, a bank teller, and a speech tutor while I formulated this plan. Unfortunately, I have never made enough from my style of writing to support myself. Teaching others to write and appreciate pop culture not only has been an interesting career choice but afforded me the time and opportunities to write.

In 1982, I entered the master's program in technical writing at Bowling Green State University (BGSU) in Ohio, where I had the kind of "adult" experiences that other students often have in high school or undergrad years at university. I fell in love, had sex, and partied, but I still managed a 4.0 grade point average. In 1983, I decided that I enjoyed being a consulting technical communicator doing freelance writing or editing but did not want to work full-time in a cubicle within a tech company. Instead, I pursued my Ph.D. in—get this—English, with specializations in rhetoric, composition, technical communication, and Victorian literature. My dissertation was about technical communication and then-new ways to use word processing on the job. At that time, BGSU did not have a Ph.D. in technical communication, so, like Sherlock Holmes creating his own job title of consulting detective, I created my own unique doctoral degree title. I, like Holmes, am the only one in the world to have such a title. By 1989, I was well on my way to being tenured at the University of Findlay, just down the road from Bowling Green.

During my career, my investment in professional associations has certainly paid off in high-profile positions within organizations. They also mark different "mini-lives" within my career. While I worked toward my M.A. and Ph.D. at BGSU, I served as editor for the newsletter produced by the student chapter of the Society for Technical Communication (STC). When I taught primarily technical communication courses at the University of Findlay and worked part-time as a consultant, I became the director of the STC chapters of Region 4 (Ohio, Indiana, Michigan, Kentucky, and Illinois) and a member of the STC's board of directors. Later I was awarded the honor of becoming a Fellow. (The awards ceremony when I received my diamond pin as a fellow is especially noteworthy because, like a true nerd, I mark the event with a pop culture memory. As I walked around downtown Toronto that day, I met actor Paul Gross, who was filming the television series *Due South* (1994–1999). Gross is one of my favorite actors, and, although I have seen him perform on stage or had the opportunity to talk with him a few times, meeting him this first time was extra special. I even got to hold his character's red Mountie coat between scenes.) Not only did positions in the STC teach me about leadership and the profession of technical communication outside of academia, but board meetings, regional chapter meetings, and conferences gave me plenty of opportunities to travel around the country and enjoy once-in-a-lifetime outside-of-work experiences.

My career path abruptly changed direction, in part, because of my parents. In 1993, Dad was diagnosed with terminal lung cancer; Mom needed some help in Florida, where they had recently retired; and I was questioning whether I "fit" as a faculty member in Findlay. During and after Dad's illness, I frequently visited Florida and ended up quitting my teaching job so I could write and "help" Mom in a warmer climate. By 2001, I had tired of part-time teaching in person or online and applied for a tenure-track position at Embry-Riddle Aeronautical University (ERAU) in Daytona Beach. I was hired, over time earned tenure again, and became a full professor—the highest-level job title I would ever achieve. I never wanted to be an administrator but preferred to be left alone to develop courses to teach and to conduct research and write.

I had enjoyed being a technical writer or editor, but, after the permanent move to Florida in 2001, I largely gave up my identity as a technical communicator. Instead, my research interests returned me to an old love—popular culture—and I participated in regional and national conferences as a member of the Popular Culture Association (PCA) and the Popular Culture Association in the South (PCAS). As a member of ERAU's Humanities and Social Sciences (later Humanities and Communication) Department, I was encouraged to pursue my pop culture interests, especially because they led to numerous presentations and publications not only around the United States but in Canada, England, Australia, and New Zealand. My PCAS participation at the annual conferences and role as a journal's associate editor prepared me for my next leadership role. Just before I was first diagnosed with cancer, I became the editor of the journal *Studies in Popular Culture.*

During my writing career, I authored or co-authored books about my pop culture favorites: television series *LOST, Battlestar Galactica, Heroes, Doctor Who/Torchwood,* and *Sherlock*; book and film series *The Lord of the Rings* and *The Hobbit*; artist Vincent van Gogh; and actor Benedict Cumberbatch. I joke that Cumberbatch bought me my last car. Granted, it was previously owned and a compact model, but I was still proud that I earned enough from my three performance biographies tracking his career to pay cash for my "new" vehicle. During this time, I also wrote articles and reviews, as well as had my own column for a couple of years in the online magazine *PopMatters.* During my parallel work as an editor across 20 years of reading others' work, I served as a proofreader of textbooks, the *Academy of Management Review,* and *The Philosopher's Index,* and as the copy editor of *The Journal of Sex Research* (not nearly as titillating as you might think) before becoming the editor of *Studies in Popular Culture.*

The focus on my career illustrates my often-workaholic nature, especially during my 30s and 40s. I seldom dated past 40 and only came to understand my lack of interest in potential lifetime partners late in life. I never married. I never had children. Instead, I enjoyed my relationships with Bart, my sister-in-law Nancy, and my niece Heather; best friends and their children, who allow me to be an honorary auntie; and colleagues who also are good friends. I have traveled almost everywhere I wanted to go and especially thrilled to adventures in Australia, New Zealand, and Belize. In Belize, for example, I (probably stupidly) held a wild howler monkey who wanted to share my lunch, first truly saw the Milky Way from a boat silently floating along a crocodile-infested river, and avoided a scorpion as big as my hand while hiking to a Mayan temple. For someone who is not athletic—or who might more appropriately be described as klutzy—I have sometimes walked far off that beaten path. I may have envisioned myself as Indiana Jones, but I can only truly claim the "Indiana" title as a result of being born a Hoosier. Most of the time my adventures are more likely to be fan based rather than action oriented.

Bolstered by information from Mom, who tracked down the deepest roots of her family tree, and DNA results provided by Ancestry.com, I honor my Scottish ancestry by attending local Highland Games as often as possible and more than once touring Scotland. On a memorable Thanksgiving break in 2011, I combined my love for Scotland and pop culture with my infatuation with actor/singer John Barrowman by flying to Glasgow for the weekend, just to see Barrowman in concert. I was fortunate to be seated across the aisle from his partner and parents, and when John Jr. asked everyone to rise, join hands, and sing "Auld Lang Syne," John Sr. took my hand and, after the song, chatted with me about, strangely enough, living in Florida, where we both resided much of the year. This is the kind of experience I often have had as a result of being a writer or a fan. Instead of long-term relationships, I have a few close familial and adoptive-family relationships and a host of brief encounters with people who have influenced me through their art.

My life is unique, but it shares commonalities with many adults around my age who grew up in the Midwest in the latter half of the 20th century. I may be "other" in several ways from my peers or colleagues, but I also did what many of us were expected to do—grow up, go to school, get a university degree, get a job, and have a family (biological or "built" over time). That cancer has become part of my story is not even that unusual these days, and, given my family's medical history, I probably should have anticipated that I would develop cancer at some point in my life. However, cancer isn't the whole story of my life, even if it's the focus of a year—perhaps the final year—in my life.

In short, as Jimmy Stewart's George Bailey discovers, no matter how dark life seems to be at times, *It's a Wonderful Life* (1946). All of my experiences—including those resulting from cancer—have made me who I am, and I am grateful for my life, no matter how it ends.

Introduction

November 1, 2018.

What could be a more fitting day than Día de los Muertos for sitting down to revisit my life and impending death as I begin this memoir? Only last night I spent Halloween looking at the Facebook photos of my friends' and their children's costumes, images that my adoptive family uploaded while trick-or-treating. I recalled that last year I joined them, a devoted auntie protecting kids from unobservant drivers, overprotective dogs, and even a bear. (A bear sighting in their Longwood, Florida, neighborhood eventually broke up our trick-or-treating trek.) I also remembered that the year before last I had been wheelchair bound on Halloween; during that autumn I underwent intravenous (IV) chemotherapy treatments. Last year I basked not only in the October warmth of a Florida Halloween but in the joy of being able to hike around the neighborhood unaided. This year, like the ghosts reportedly hovering between this world and the next, I am in limbo between being a recent cancer patient cautious about feeling cured and a woman with a terminal diagnosis. Therefore, this year when I stopped clicking through the Halloween photos, I ended my evening more spiritually than by eating chocolate pilfered from one of the children's bags. My solitary Samhain celebration included a meditation in front of rows of candles on the hearth and a harvest feast of apples, almonds, and wine. I am growing less active and more meditative during the symbolic autumn of my life, and I can't help but wonder if next year I will join the multicultural harvest festivities as a corporeal reveler or a remembered spirit. Will I celebrate Día de los Muertos or be one of the celebrated?

In April 2016, I was diagnosed with colorectal cancer. After weeks of chemotherapy and radiation, in August I had surgery to remove a cancerous rectal tumor. As part of the cancer surgery, I was given a temporary ileostomy, which was reversed in March 2017. However, I still suffer the consequences of my life-saving surgery by daily trying to placate an unpredictable, often embarrassing digestive system. Between these surgeries, I endured months of IV chemotherapy via a port that had been installed in my chest during a brief outpatient surgery. During autumn 2016, I often felt like a pod person in a bad science fiction film. In a mostly silent room in a cancer center, I sat in a recliner for hours as one of the dozens of patients tethered to chemo bags hung on poles, all of us watching the life-prolonging poison drip into our veins.

Possibly as a result of chemotherapy, a half dozen blood clots managed to travel through my body to land in my lungs. On the day I could barely breathe or walk into the appointment with my oncologist, he immediately sent me to a nearby clinic for a series of scans. They showed more deep vein thromboses (DVTs) ready to journey from legs to lungs to join the pulmonary embolisms (PEs) already there. For six months I took medication to dissolve the clots and, for once in my life, had a legitimate reason to sit as quietly as possible and watch television all day. While I was on chemo, my eyesight also changed drastically every few weeks; I needed new glasses six times in eight months. My cataracts grew, and, in August 2017, I underwent eye surgeries for glaucoma and clouded lenses. Metal stents helped relieve the pressure caused by glaucoma, and artificial lenses replaced the hardened disks in my eyes.

Nevertheless, I felt all the frustration, fear, and pain of these treatments and surgeries had been worth it. Shortly after my IV chemo treatments ended, my scans looked positive. The carcinoembryonic antigen (CEA) level is often the tumor marker or biomarker used to help diagnose colorectal cancer or, if the cancer returns after surgery or treatment, to guide a prognosis. As one oncology website explains, a decrease in the tumor-marker number may be positive, indicating that the cancer is responding to treatment. If the tumor marker doesn't change or, worse, the number increases, the treatment may not be working, or cancer may have returned (OncoLink Team). True to its medical definition, my tumor marker confidently predicted my disease. Along with the extremely negative (as in "bad," unfortunately not as in "no cancer") results of my colonoscopy and follow-up scans, my first biomarker number was 17, well over the 10 that is a usually accurate indication of cancer. (Anything above 5 is cause for a lot of concern.) My CEA tests during chemo showed that the number was steadily dropping during treatments. After my last treatment, I scored a 2 in January 2017—a great way to start the year. No one scores a 0, so my measly 2 was respectable and encouraging. I left the cancer institute with hope, as well as an enduring fear of needles. As soon as possible, I underwent the ileostomy reversal and, a month later, had the port removed.

I was determined to succeed as a cancer survivor. After all, friends or parents of friends went through similar diagnoses and treatments and were cancer free years later. Yet, I always knew that success or failure is not a useful way of thinking of having cancer. As far as anyone can tell, getting cancer wasn't my fault; my behavior wasn't risky, such as years of smoking making lung cancer more of a possibility. Going along with doctors' recommended treatments and surgeries, if they worked, also couldn't give me the credit for successfully eliminating cancer cells and defying their return. If I don't accept blame for having cancer, then I can't take the credit for remaining cancer free. Nonetheless, I really wanted to be one of those cancer survivors.

In late July, my follow-up blood work indicated my latest cancer-marker score was 5—the tipping point between "normal" and "likely having cancer." So I began to worry as I returned to teaching in autumn 2017. I felt healthy, but "the number" continually lurked in the dark corners of my mind.

In January 2018, my regularly scheduled follow-up scans confirmed that cancer had metastasized in my lungs. These were ambitious little cancer cells, too. They settled at Stage 4—inoperable and untreatable. My oncologist said my CEA score might increase exponentially as the tumors grow larger. When asked if I wanted a port again and more chemo, possibly to prolong my life a few weeks, I declined. I may not have years or even months to live, but I will not live them connected to a chemo bag. My days as a pod person are over, even if that means my days are over even sooner—period. My choice is not what others, even in my family, have made. Bart, for example, participated in every test, said yes to every experimental surgery, and took chemo throughout the remainder of his life—all to spend as much time as possible with his family. I choose to spend time alternating between living as healthfully as possible and indulging my taste for chocolate or Hollandaise sauce. I am now terminal, but that does not mean I stop living.

Such is the life of a dead woman—or one who is dying openly and faster than she expected. Those who are diagnosed with a terminal disease and given a short time to live are often considered by the rest of the population as already dead. Unless forced to confront our death, most of us are content to ignore mortality, and being or being around terminally ill patients can be mentally and emotionally taxing—for the cared-for and the caregivers. The terminally ill have entered a unique realm of living—here but soon not-to-be-here.

Living with a terminal diagnosis is akin to becoming a zombie. Since I watched the movie *Cargo* (2017), I can more readily relate to Martin Freeman's Andy, whose wife is attacked by a zombie. During her transformation, she bites her husband. Andy knows that he will soon become a zombie, too, but he has 48 hours in which to find someone to look after his infant daughter. Like Andy, who attempted to circumvent death-by-zombie by carefully navigating a river to a safe haven, I was aware of potential dangers (i.e., cancer running through my family) as I navigated my life journey. Yet, Andy and I both were surprised when deadly danger ambushed us. Like Andy, I watched in horror and helplessness as my family was fatally stricken. Andy lost his wife; I lost my paternal grandparents, maternal grandmother, father, and brother. Like Andy, I was "bitten" by the same ailment that took my family and, in a short period of time, decided on a plan to protect those left behind (e.g., Andy finds a home for his daughter; I set up a trust for those closest to me). In the end, I hope I am still relating to Andy, who knows what to do so as not to hurt others when he becomes incapacitated and ultimately finds a measure of grace in a gruesome, too-early demise.

Yet, despite living in my personal zombie movie, I also frequently remind myself that physicist, author, and celebrity Stephen Hawking was diagnosed with amyotrophic lateral sclerosis (ALS) in 1963 and told to expect to live only a couple of years at most. That prognosis proved to be inaccurate; Hawking died in 2018 (Ryan). I can't rely on such an outcome for myself, but stories like Hawking's illustrate miraculous ways in which a body can surprise medical science.

A potential problem with doctors who work with terminally ill patients is their scientifically founded preconceptions about the progression of a disease. For example, an often-cited 2009 article in the National Institutes of Health's U.S. National Library of Medicine, "Surgical Management of Colorectal Lung Metastasis," provides a depressingly low percentage of people who live with Stage 4 (metastasized) colorectal cancer, "an extremely prevalent cancer, with greater than 1 million cases identified in the world yearly. Of these cases, 19% present with stage IV disease.... Overall survival with untreated stage IV disease is 11.3% at 5 years" (Villeneuve and Sundaresan). The authors indicate that resection of the lung, the second most common site of metastasized colorectal cancer, increases the patient's lifespan. My tumors are spread throughout both lungs, and surgical removal of some or all tumors is not an option. Thus, maybe I could possibly, luckily be part of that 11.3 percent four or more years from now, but I won't bet my future on it. Although medical breakthroughs or new technologies are gradually increasing the likelihood that cancer can be detected earlier and/or treated more effectively, the survival rate for my type of cancer really has not increased that much since this article was published in 2009.

Doctors may admit they can't guarantee a prognosis; a patient's life may be shorter or longer than is typically expected. However, they have access to a wide range of data about, as well as vast professional experience with typical disease progression. Patients, their friends, and their family likely form their ideas about what is going to happen based on more than the scientific knowledge provided by doctors; their preconceptions are just as likely to be formed by anecdotal information from friends and colleagues, personal experiences, or the influence of popular culture representations of a specific disease.

A combination of medical and anecdotal evidence of what the progression of metastatic bowel cancer may be like helped me compare my expectations about dying of Stage 4 rectal cancer that, so far, has metastasized to my lungs with similar patients' attitudes and experiences. The 2017 article "Living and Dying with Metastatic Bowel Cancer: Serial In-Depth Interviews with Patients" resulted from a series of three interviews with terminally ill bowel cancer patients in the U.K. soon after their diagnosis, during the period when they could still live a relatively "normal" life, and when they were very near the end of their lives.

Three findings particularly stood out to me. Soon after a terminal diagnosis, the studied group "were uncertain about how the illness would progress and what their future would hold, even hoping they may avoid their likely fate. However, some participants had started planning for dying with their relatives" (Carduff, Kendall, and Murray). Perhaps I am just a fatalist, but, when presented with a terminal diagnosis, I immediately accepted I was going to die and almost as quickly started thinking of what I needed to accomplish before I did. I focused as much on the "business of dying" as any bucket-list leisure plans. Like the patients interviewed for this study, I was primarily curious how and how fast the cancer would progress. More than a year after my diagnosis, I still don't know what to expect when.

Bart, more than I, could relate to those interviewees who "wanted to know that their lives had been meaningful" (Carduff, Kendall, and Murray). Maybe because he, like the majority of the study's participants, had a family who relied on him, he and these interviewees were very much concerned about their legacy. Although my concern with a legacy comes and goes, I hope that my loved ones have some pleasant memories of me and will think of me once I am gone. Because I don't have traditional "legacy markers" such as a career noted for changing society or discovering something new, or more common socio-biological accomplishments such as bearing children, my legacy is ultimately determined by the people who know me best. I agreed most with those research participants who "expressed concern about what material ... legacy they were leaving their families" (Carduff, Kendall, and Murray). Assessing my finances and trying to determine how much money I will need for the rest of my life and how and how much wealth to distribute to family and friends have become a key focus in my dying days.

My greatest concern during my first, perhaps only year as a "dead" woman is anxiety about dependency and social isolation as a result of my impending and unavoidable physical deterioration while my healthy cells succumb to cancer. Again, like these research participants, I "desire to maintain a semblance of normality in [my life], but illness progression made this increasingly difficult" (Carduff, Kendall, and Murray). Being unable to work or socialize "normally," becoming a burden on those closest to me, and losing my identity or "normal" self because of disease are, I have come to understand, perfectly normal concerns for "dead" people like me.

Although these findings provided a scientific determination of how

I measure up to others facing similar end-of-life physical, psychological, and emotional issues, I found the way that two participants, Ian and Andrew, faced their prognosis to be most instructive. Ian received a two-year prognosis; after 18 months, he thought that he was approaching the end. Andrew had not been given a specific prognosis; instead of anticipating his lifespan in months, he set personal goals or chose events that he wanted to attend (Carduff, Kendall, and Murray). My prognosis experience falls somewhere between Ian's and Andrew's. Initially I was given a six-month to one-year prognosis, but that was later expanded, and, as I write this memoir, I have no idea of how many more days, weeks, months, or years oncologists expect me to live, much less how much more time I really have. I assume fewer rather than more months, but, like Andrew, I try to set goals, even if someday I will not be able to achieve them.

No one knows for sure what is going to happen when, and even a scientific prognosis may be misleading. The bottom line is that death will occur. Unless something else mortally wounds the body first, the cancer cells overcome healthy cells and lead to death.

Thus, as one of the living dead, I am unsure how to realistically or how long to plan future activities, on the job or on vacation. As a still-fully-employed professor, I am unsure how to regard my future teaching schedule or give hints to my employer about the likelihood of my continuing to work. At some point before the typical retirement age, I will be unable to teach my classes because I am disabled or dead. Because course schedules and faculty workloads are planned about a year in advance, when is it logical for my name no longer to appear on a schedule? How soon is too soon to begin planning to file for disability, to retire early, or to die? When I want to enjoy time away from my career, making plans creates another level of anxiety. If I decide to make plans months in advance, I worry that I may not be around when it's time to take a trip or attend an event. Yet, if I don't make plans, I fear that I'm missing out on life, because someday I may be stuck at home or in a hospital. When I talk with a travel agent about a cruise I want to take, I'm informed that I should have either planned a year or more ago or should book a cruise currently a year or more hence. I then must explain why "sooner," such as in the next month or two, may be my only option. My urgency then engenders pity or horror. After all, who wants to think that waiting until next week for a booking to be confirmed or next month to take a cruise may be too late?

For the terminally ill, life is paradoxically certain (e.g., Death-by-cancer is going to happen) and uncertain (e.g., Will medications be readily available to eliminate pain? Should I retire now or hang in there at work until the last minute? Do I have time to do whatever is top priority? Will something else get me first?). Life becomes the clichéd litany of everything matters and nothing matters. However, such uncertainty and contradictions are the nature of life for everyone, not just the terminally ill. Those who have been diagnosed with a terminal illness simply have the luxury of becoming acutely aware of life's paradox. Everyone will die of something someday. Having a more likely idea of how or when can be a burden or a blessing. I choose to feel blessed and take advantage of the time I have been given. Like *Cargo*'s Andy, I use the knowledge that I am dying in order to take care of the business of life, especially by looking after my loved ones.

Dealing with others' preconceptions about dying, however, is as difficult for me as the process of dying. When I cleared out my condo of the unnecessary "stuff" with which most of us clutter our homes, I chatted with the young man conscientiously carrying boxes and bags downstairs to his truck, which he drove numerous times to donation sites or a landfill.

"I want to make sure that my house is clean and ready for my niece," I casually remarked as he struggled with yet another box of books to be donated. "Are you moving?" he asked. "Is that why you're getting rid of so much stuff?" I hesitated before honestly confessing, "I've been given only a few months to live. I don't want my niece to have to go through all my junk and figure out what to do with everything." He stopped and stared at me. "But you seem so happy." His response was similar to that of many people I encounter. My calm, pragmatic demeanor did not mesh with his preconception of someone with a death sentence.

A trip to the dentist for a six-month cleaning and check-up led to another typical response: inspiration. The routine question "Any changes to your health?" received a blunt answer: "Yes, the cancer has returned, and I've been told I have six months." After a stunned silence, the dental hygienist asked if I was receiving chemo and needed my oncologist's permission to have my teeth cleaned. (For insurance reasons, many dentists require signed permission forms from doctors treating cancer patients before an invasive treatment can be given.) "Nope," I replied. "I'm not going to have any treatments. Nothing can be done at this point." The hygienist took a deep breath. "Do you want x-rays?" This time I grinned. "I'm not particularly fond of any more radiation, so I'll take my chances with cavities." She smiled back, made notes, and cleaned my teeth. As she removed the bib I wore during the cleaning, she said, "You seem so relaxed today. I wouldn't know you have cancer." A few minutes later she returned with the dentist, who asked how I was doing and admitted he had been told about my situation. "I'm having a great time, actually," I enthused. "I'm going to Iceland in a few weeks. I've never been there but always wanted to go." The dentist hugged me and told me I had made his day—in fact, I was inspirational. Not quite knowing what to say, I thanked him and determinedly walked to the front desk to make my next six-month appointment.

Apparently, the dying are not supposed to embody joy or look outwardly healthy, especially while giving away their worldly possessions or having their teeth polished. Dancing around my bedroom to Pharrell Williams singing "Happy" seems inconceivable to normal people. Of course, I want to live as long and healthfully as possible. However, I choose to enjoy the sun's warmth on my face, a rich first cup of morning coffee, or a dear friend's hug instead of worrying how many minutes/hours/days/weeks I might be around to savor these simple gifts or how horribly I might suffer before I give up.

Dealing with others' concepts of what is "appropriate" to say or do as a dying person is an area with which I often struggle. Fortunately, those who know me best accept my irreverent dark humor. When my department chair, Sally Blomstrom, heard that, about 10 months past my terminal diagnosis, I planned to spend the upcoming months writing books, she enthusiastically congratulated me but worried about my being overwhelmed with teaching and other professional responsibilities. "I'm concerned about your schedule," she solemnly said. "I know," I replied. "I hope it doesn't kill me." Sally paused only a second before her deadpan response: "That's funny. You should write that down." (See, Sally. I did.)

As I have always done, I turn to popular culture as a resource for the evolution of my philosophy of life and death. My favorite films and television series helpfully provide visuals with which to compare my dying with the dramatized process of others. A song lyric or a line of dialogue may stand out all of a sudden and have an entirely new meaning for me than it would have had before my initial cancer diagnosis, even if that personal meaning is wildly out of its "correct" context. For me, popular culture is one way of making the abstract concept of death more specific and of using fiction to help come to terms with my reality.

Strangely enough, one of the most annoying aspects of a terminal diagnosis and a short shelf life is my love of serialized fiction or films. Bart, after seeing the second installment of Peter Jackson's *Hobbit* trilogy, *The Desolation of Smaug* (2013), pensively watched the credits roll and wondered aloud if he would be alive to see the final film the following year. Like Bart, I now need to carefully choose which films are best to see in the time I have left. Even while I remain relatively healthy, I also must consider whether my post-surgery, post-treatment body can handle a multi-hour excursion that day. A simple trip to the cinema can have emotional and physical consequences. I have to decide if or what to eat or drink and how the film's run time might affect my ability to stay seated through the closing credits and their "tags," the extra scenes providing clues to future films. My digestive system might "explode" with little warning—at least causing me to miss a key plot point as I sprint to the restroom and, at most, leading to public embarrassment. Then, if I decide to venture to the cinema, I have the critical choice of what to see. With hindsight, cliffhangers such as *Avengers: Infinity War* (2018) and *Fantastic Beasts: The Crimes of Grindelwald* (2018) may not have been good choices, given that their concluding sequels may be released months or years after my demise. However, even these frustrating film choices ultimately have paid off by adding to my understanding of favorite characters or even helping to illustrate my philosophy of life and death.

During a *Tonight Show* interview in November 2018, actor Benedict Cumberbatch discussed the fate of his Marvelverse character, Doctor Strange, who, near the end of *Avengers: Infinity War*, disintegrates at a snap of uber-villain Thanos' (Josh Brolin) fingers. The good doctor had previously traveled through time to study all possible outcomes of the Avengers' and other superheroes' war to stop Thanos, but only the outcome in which half of the universe's population dies could possibly lead to ultimate victory over the infinity stones-wielding conqueror. Before filmgoers' eyes, Strange becomes dust in the wind. When *Tonight Show* host Jimmy Fallon asked Cumberbatch about his character's fate, the actor exclaimed, "I'm dust, baby. I'm just out there ... in the ether" (Mitchell).

I like that description, which is close to my expectation of what will happen to my body upon its death. This image is one reason why I toy with the idea of having Kansas' "Dust in the Wind" (1977) and Queen's "Another One Bites the Dust" (1980) played at my memorial get-together.

I believe that my energy as Lynnette Raye Porter simply will take another form. Quite practically, my cremated body will become ashes to be scattered on a beach or entombed in the family plot. The First Law of Thermodynamics can be simplified in a comforting philosophical way as "energy can be converted from one form to another …, but it **cannot** [original emphasis] be created nor destroyed, under any circumstances" (LibreTexts Project). As a pop culture enthusiast, I envision this law in action as Doctor Strange flaking away. (Perhaps I am merely flaky because I value this illustration of death.) Like Doctor Strange, I soon may be in the ether.

However, I choose not to accept Cumberbatch's follow-up comment that Strange's "dust" is probably part of the food chain and may be gurgling through our stomachs. That image is a bit too *Soylent Green* (1973) for me, even as a student of pop culture. ("Soylent green," the government-manufactured food for humans living on a dystopic future earth, turns out—spoiler alert—to be made from deceased people. "Soylent green is people!" an agonized Charlton Heston [as Detective Frank Thorn] exclaims, giving the movie its most memorable line.)

More positively than the *Soylent Green* imagery, the following documentaries and a mainstream film, all released in 2018—the year of my terminal diagnosis—unexpectedly led me to think more seriously about my life experiences and the cultural impact of a single life.

• Academy Award-winning *Free Solo* explores the solitary life of freestyle mountain climber Alex Honnold, whose solo climb of Yosemite's El Capitan is immortalized on film. Like Honnold, I am often solitary in my lifestyle, despite having the support of friends and family. Some of those who love me, however, can't understand the risks I take with my life, and they expend a great deal of energy in trying to change my philosophy or behavior. To those who want me to continue chemo, get a second (third, fourth, fifth) medical opinion, or retire to rest in the comfort of my home, I must seem like a solo climber undertaking a dangerous ascent toward the heavens, knowing that any misstep can result in a hellish plummet. However, this "climb" is one I must make on my own terms, as Honnold did. Instead, well-wishers who are not facing a solo climb would prefer that Honnold or I keep both feet solidly on the ground and do what is expected of us, that is, act normally.

In the months after hearing my prognosis, I began to undertake as many bucket-list trips as possible, and I often travel solo. First, I flew to Iceland and visited remote, frigid landscapes of immense beauty where I could stand above foaming waterfalls or feel (and smell) the sulfuric spray of a geyser. Weeks later, I wandered New Orleans' French Quarter to hear late-night jazz in clubs and on the streets. Next, I dared to fly non-stop to Copenhagen (a true test of courage, given my ongoing digestive problems) to spend a day at nearby "Hamlet's castle" (Kronborg) before embarking on a cruise around Scandinavia. When I first learned of my cancer, I decided that Kronborg would be close to the top of my travel priorities because *Hamlet* is my favorite Shakespearean play. Before my surgery, I even toyed with the notion of flying to Copenhagen just to take the train to the castle. Three years later, I finally fulfilled my wish to spend a whole day touring the castle on my own. Running into (actors playing) Hamlet and Ophelia in a hallway gallery and overhearing their argument over Hamlet's love letters and, later, in the throne room witnessing fencing only a few feet away more than fulfilled my wish to visit Hamlet's home. A few weeks after my return from Europe, I made the first of two trips to New Mexico. In Albuquerque I rented a sedan (with hindsight, not the best choice of off-road vehicle) and bounced along pitted dirt roads or within rutted truck tracks to the base of Ship Rock or into Chaco Canyon—places where my phone could not receive a signal and no one (including, at times, me) knew my exact whereabouts. Being a solo senior traveler suffering from the effects of previous surgeries and an uncertain medical future seemed, at least to some people, as daunting as climbing hand over hand up the face of El Capitan, especially when I felt adventuresome and overly confident of my ability to always come home safely.

• Another documentary, *Love, Gilda*, celebrates the life of original *Saturday Night Live* cast member Gilda Radner, who died of ovarian cancer. Instead of writing a line like "Unfortunately, she is now best known for the manner of her death," I, like the documentarists who chronicled her life, relish the way that she turned her termination notice into a source of comedy. I remember her last television appearance on *It's Garry Shandling's Show* in 1988, a feisty performance replayed in the documentary. When Shandling introduces Radner to the studio audience, the crowd cheers, and she exuberantly raises her arms in triumph. Shandling then asks why she has been absent from television. "I had cancer," Radner chirps—destigmatizing a scene that plays out too often in the lives of cancer patients (through well-meaning questions like "What happened to you?," "Why weren't you at [fill in event]?," or "Where have you been?" The answer often results in a pitying smile or worried frown). Gilda being Gilda, she then asks Shandling, "What did you have?" Shandling, being self-deprecatory Shandling, replies that his primetime absence was due to bad career decisions.

Upon reflecting on the documentary and my unexpectedly emotional reaction to it, I posted this almost-coming-out-as-terminally-ill message on my Facebook page.

> At 14, I crushed on Gene Wilder; at 18, "SNL"'s Gilda Radner. On my own for the first time in September 1975, I fervently watched "SNL" each week; it opened a new world of possibilities—of comedy, of creativity, of a city like New York. And Gilda Radner played with such joy and abandon. I faithfully returned to "SNL" every Saturday night for the five seasons of Gilda. When she and Wilder married, they became my dream team of comedy and romance—a real-life rom-com, heavy on the rom—even if their films together didn't live up to my (or most critics') expectations. However, their greatest gift to me was the way they tackled Gilda's cancer together. Back then, I had only lost one person to cancer, but I learned by Gilda's public example. "Love, Gilda" let me laugh out loud again at Emily Litella and be inspired by the woman who wanted "She had a good time" on her tombstone. If you're old enough to have enjoyed Gilda on "SNL," you probably will enjoy seeing favorite characters once more, and the bio may be a revelation. But if you're someone with cancer or you love someone with cancer, the film

brings recognition of, but never suggests resignation to, being a member of Gilda's Club [the nationwide cancer-support organization Radner founded]; it's a reminder that love and laughter are the point of life [September 21, 2018, post].

Gilda Radner, through her performances and comments replayed in *Love, Gilda*, makes me want to emulate her spirit.

• The mainstream film *Bohemian Rhapsody*, primarily a biopic of Queen's lead singer, Freddie Mercury, also struck a chord, not only because Mercury succumbed to then-incurable AIDS but because he celebrated otherness. I first became aware of Queen in the mid–1970s, when I turned up the radio every morning during the drive from my very first apartment to classes at then–Indiana State University–Evansville (ISUE) and heard "We Are the Champions" (1975) or "Somebody to Love" (1976). My parents and brother moved to Ohio between my high school graduation and the start of my first year as an undergraduate student, and I reveled in the freedom of my first apartment. Especially during my undergraduate years, I struggled to find out who I was or was going to be. I strove to be "other" from the introverted, sheltered high school scholar. I had always been a good student: I earned a full academic scholarship to study history at ISUE. Testing my independence and feeling unexpectedly rebellious, I quickly determined that I could attend one of every six Monday-Wednesday-Friday classes (the required minimum to stay enrolled in a course) and still maintain straight A's. (I don't recommend this approach to my students.) When I didn't attend my classes, I sat in on my best friend Genie Horn's classes or spent the day at the zoo. My out-of-class undergraduate education later included performing in plays (I wouldn't term it "acting"), exploring the new academic area of radio/television/film studies, spending afternoons at the movies, and trying to understand why I had little desire to date men (who seemed intimidated or uninterested in asking me out anyway). Queen provided my first inkling of what it means to be "other." I was, and am, different in many ways from my peers—a fact which I celebrated and embraced decades later while watching *Bohemian Rhapsody*. Seeing Oscar-winner Rami Malek (who also attended university—U of Evansville—in my hometown) inhabit the role of Freddie Mercury, especially as he deals with his AIDS diagnosis, only cemented Queen's continuing influence in my life and reminded me of my long-ago pop culture "mentor" who was unafraid to be himself.

I realize that two of the three most recent films that resonate with my life post-death diagnosis glorify famous people who have died of terrible diseases. Oddly enough, I share common ground with such famous people as Gilda Radner or Freddie Mercury; we all lived with the understanding that a deadly disease will have its cavalier way with our body. Yet, I also believe our commonalities include tenacity, love of the moment, and a desire to share our life experiences—bad or good—with the whole world.

I don't delude myself into believing that I could ever be as well known or influential as these talented celebrities or that I will be remembered in history. Instead, I have enjoyed meeting and, whenever possible, interviewing or just chatting with those whose names likely will be remembered for years to come. I am attracted to creative people who tell stories, whether they write, act, or direct them, because stories—fact or fiction—make the human experience comprehensible and meaningful. By engaging with people in the entertainment industry as a fan-scholar, I learn how and why inspirational stories are made and why and how certain characters have become important examples of how to deal with the struggles inherent in life or death. Whom we choose to immortalize on film and why we are fascinated with famous people who have died of an incurable disease reflect the way we, as a society, think of death and those who are dying.

Like many people who go to the movies or follow the lives of celebrities, I believed the fiction (or fictionalized depictions of facts) related to death and dying. My preconceptions about dying were formed as much by popular culture as by my interactions with dying family members. Now that I am one of the "walking dead," I more clearly understand what it is like to deal with others' preconceptions about what is expected from the death process or even considered socially appropriate behavior from the terminally ill. Although, in this book, I am a case study of one—hardly a scientific sample—I hope that sharing my story of living with a terminal cancer diagnosis and confronting my and others' expectations about life and death with cancer will provide insights into the dissonance between the popularized fiction or fantasy of dying and the reality of coming to grips with one's mortality.

CHAPTER 1

Living the Dream/
Fearing the Wake-up Call

If I am going to bury my head in the sand, Papa'iloa Beach on Oahu in Hawaii is where I want to do it.

Oahu has always been a special place for me—first, in early 2007, as a stopover to discuss J. R. R. Tolkien's *The Lord of the Rings* with the Tolkien Society on my way from the mainland to a sabbatical in New Zealand. Several times afterward, I undertook research about the television series *LOST* (2004–2010), which was filmed all around the island, or to present papers about popular culture at the Hawaiian International Conference on the Arts and Humanities (HICAH) in Honolulu. Oahu is a refuge when real life becomes too much and I choose to bask in the fantasy of life on a tropical island.

Although I had finished taking chemotherapy in December 2016 and showed no signs of cancer in my January 2017 scans, I still felt far from carefree. Summer and autumn 2017 left my emotions exhausted after the careening highs and lows better suited for an Orlando theme park. In late July 2017, I received frightening indications from my "cancer marker" tests (resulting emotion: anxiety with a chaser of fear). I fared much better with successful eye surgeries in August (emotion: relief that I am not blind! and can travel in a few months!). In mid–August, I started the academic year by teaching classes with students I could not see more than two feet beyond my nose; however, Antonia Santacroce, a compassionate and efficient student assistant, led me to and from the classroom and kept a sharp eye on my students when they were just blurs with voices to me. My emotions veered from day to day: joy that I would see better after lens replacements and stent implants tempered by frustration that my eyes required more than a month to

27

heal; relief that I could still hold a job, despite my many surgeries and physical setbacks in the past 18 months; and anxiety at the realization I would always have post-cancer surgical problems. My outward scars were minimal dents in my skin, but the important wounds to my ego and self-esteem scarred jaggedly. After one conversation in which I defensively tried to explain the reasons why I failed to notice some key content problems in an article I edited, my exasperated co-editor said, "You cannot be that insecure." She relied on her experiences with "past me"—the confident, secure professor and editor relied upon to mentor junior faculty and guide novice authors. The post-past me is new but not improved and trying desperately to pass for emotionally steady, professionally reliable, and physically on par with the woman I was about 10 years ago. The upcoming getaway to Oahu could not come soon enough.

My next challenge, in September, was a solo drive across Florida's panhandle with one eye patched as I escaped the imminent wrath of Hurricane Matthew (emotions: anxiety from wondering how my near-beachside condo would fare, relief from being out of the storm's immediate path, and strangely proud that I could take care of myself). Yarggh, mateys, I might look like a castoff from a bad pirate movie, and my timbers might be shivered, but I was not blown away by Matthew or limited eyesight.

Thus, by January 2018, I felt independent enough to begin traveling farther from home and coming closer to being the (I hope respected) professor/author I had been prior to cancer. At least, I was keeping up appearances. However, I felt equally and paradoxically dependent on strangers who could either make my journeys and work life easier or so difficult that I did not know some days if I would be able to return home and, once there, if I could leave the house again.

Shortly after the new year, I felt more than eager to return to Oahu for a research-and-writing trip based at the Turtle Bay Resort on North Shore and an academic conference (HICAH), where I would present two papers at the Hilton Hawaiian Village convention center. (As I have often told my thesis students, pick your research topics carefully. Popular culture and my book projects about television series or films have brought me to Oahu six times.)

After flight delays, a long line at the car rental counter, and a traffic jam rendering the lone main road circling North Shore nearly impassable as I inched toward Turtle Bay, at sunset I arrived at my destination. I hurriedly unpacked so that I could enjoy taco night on the hotel's patio. There, I kicked back and listened to a singer croon two of my "Hawaiian memories" songs from previous trips: Israel (Iz) Kamakawiwo'ole's "Somewhere Over the Rainbow/What a Wonderful World" (1990) and Oasis' "Wonderwall" (1995).

In 2007, I heard Iz music almost all the time I cruised back and forth between my rented room in Kailua and the Kualoa Ranch, Byodo-In Temple, and other *LOST* filming sites—including the castaways' beach camp on Papa'iloa Beach. The happy tunes set the tone for my sabbatical trips, starting in Hawaii and continuing in New Zealand, where I planned to visit film archives and filming locations. Just before I boarded my flight away from Hawaii, I teared up when I heard "Somewhere Over the Rainbow/What a Wonderful World" one last time; I quickly had learned to love Oahu and wished I could've stayed longer. (My tears would have fallen if I had not been headed to New Zealand, another of my favorite places.)

The Oasis reference is a bit more convoluted but still *LOST* related. My favorite character is Charlie Pace (Dominic Monaghan)—a heroin addict and former rock star unable to leave behind his Catholic upbringing and desire to do something redemptively good. In the episode "Flashes Before Your Eyes," Charlie plays "Wonderwall" in a flashback to his busker days, and Charlie and older brother Liam's band, Drive Shaft, was reportedly a nod to Noel and Liam Gallagher's band, Oasis.

With that symbolic and personally meaningful musical welcome back to Oahu, I sat back to enjoy the ukulele-playing singer, fish tacos, and two-for-one mai tais. About 20 minutes into my paradisiacal evening, my body betrayed me. I ran from the table to the nearest restroom, hastily assuring my server that I was not a dine-and-dash. By then, after nearly a year post-ileostomy reversal, I could interpret my scat as expertly as any jungle tracker going after big game. I read trouble in the shape and color of my waste, as well as the ferocity of my attack. However, I disposed of my fear just as efficiently as I disposed of the antiseptic-scented baggie shrouding the well-used Depends, burying both in the bottom of the restroom's trash bin. Then I nonchalantly sauntered back to my table and ordered my second mai tai. For the next

10 days, that approach helped me deal with the increasing heaviness of impending doom in what otherwise turned out to be a rewarding escape from reality.

On the way to Papa'iloa Beach the next day, I ignored the vandalism-warning signs (designed primarily to deter tourists from parking illegally along the neighborhood's dead-end road) and left my rental car close to the walkway between houses fronting the beach. One of my favorite trees from the *LOST* days guards the entrance to the beach. Its gnarly above-sand roots made the trunk seem likely to topple toward the waves back in '07. In 2018, I was pleased to see that not only had the tree survived but fuzzy green branches had begun to protrude from its root line. That weathered old tree became an inspiration. Maybe its tenacity and regrowth could prompt the same in me.

Papa'iloa beach itself has vastly changed from its *LOST* days. Then guards patrolled the orange-fenced "castaways' campsite" and the nearby site where Charlie's and Mr. Eko's (Adewale Akinnuoye-Agbaje) tied-together tree branches outlined the structure of a potential church. Of course, the remnants from filming are long gone (except from my memories and hundreds of photos). The landscape has changed in other ways, too. The sand has retreated, leaving more black rock exposed to the crashing waves. Nonetheless, this spot is sacred to me, and I meditated for at least an hour in solitude on the sand, facing the breakers. Years earlier I brought my great friend Jen Wojton to this special place. To make the day even more special, a passing offshore shower created one of Hawaii's famous rainbows, just for us. Drawing strength and peace from Papa'iloa—the television fantasy and the reality of past visits—provided an emotional touchstone for this trip.

I also returned to my roots—beyond those of the sentinel tree—by going horseback riding at Kualoa Ranch, where *LOST*, as well as more recent movies and television episodes, have been filmed. Although riding in the almost nose-to-tail line of horses was hardly equestrianly challenging, I still felt the accomplishment of being on a horse once again. When I was three, Dad led me on a tall chestnut horse with a white blaze, holding the reins and walking along a trail at Cumberland Falls State Park (now Resort Park) in Kentucky. Old Lightning and I enjoyed many a trail ride, my legs sticking almost straight out from the Western saddle as I held onto the horn. When I was 10, I rode on my own around the fenced acreage of Dad's friend's farm—until the borrowed horse decided to gallop to the barn, and I tumbled off. Pride bruised more than my butt, I learned that, when I fall off, I have to get back on that horse. When I was in graduate school in Bowling Green, Ohio, I traded hours of grooming and saddling horses for others' rides around a farm in exchange for free riding time. However, until this visit to the Kualoa Ranch, I hadn't ridden for years. Despite being content simply to ride in a supervised line, I thoroughly enjoyed the trot down memory lane.

Another tour of the ranch—this time seated on a bench in a canvas-covered truck—reminded me to enjoy the elation of the moment. After a beauty-inspired drive (with photo stops) along gently rising roads to an overlook of an ancient fish pond and the sapphire glory of the Pacific caressing the coast, our driver cautioned us to buckle up and hold on for the ride downhill. To the blaring Indiana Jones theme, the accelerating truck bounced along the rutted road. Sitting in the front row, with wind in my face and hero music in my ears, I felt wildly alive. The speed, the scenery whizzing past, and the illusion of being an Indiana Jones in Kualoa's jungle created the fantasy of starring in one of the many action movies filmed at the ranch. More important, it gave me the empowering sense that I could do anything. *That* was a perfect afternoon.

Enriching, too, were mornings in one of the Turtle Bay hot tubs overlooking the bay. Even in Hawaii, January mornings are cool, and being the first in the hot tub at 8:00 each day gave me time to soak up the warmth before the sun arrived over the mountain. I gave thanks for being able to lounge in hot water while watching the Pacific roll toward the resort and palm trees wave to the peekaboo sun. Peace, contentment, and solitude helped quell the niggling fear that all this health and harmony would soon evaporate.

When I strolled into the Waimea Valley and trudged up the hills before descending to the waterfall, I felt powerful remembering that only months earlier I couldn't walk so far, much less up or down hills, on my own. Waimea is one of those mysterious, sacred places where the flora (especially the weirdly shaped, colorful ginger plants and oversized hibiscus blossoms) and timeless shadowy valley off the paved path let visitors know there is more to life than what can be seen in the Hawaiian sunshine.

All too soon, I packed up my rental, returned it to the airport, and filed into a shuttle heading into Waikiki. Now the "work" part of my journey began. Although I kept a journal, edited articles for *Studies in Popular Culture*, and dutifully responded to work email while at Turtle Bay, I shifted from holiday visitor to professional teacher/writer the minute I picked up my room key at the Hilton Hawaiian Village and, an hour later, grabbed my conference schedule at registration. The conference was a personal triumph, reminding me that, to those who didn't know me beyond networking at the conference or hearing my presentations, I still came across as competent and confident. To other conference-goers, I seemed normal.

Not only did my conference papers go well, but I was invited to become a guest speaker at a Midwestern university as a result of one presentation. During the conference, I was in fine (if escapist) form. I networked and handed out business cards. I talked with prospective authors of journal articles. I kept up with my students back home, who had just begun a new semester a day prior to my presentations. HICAH 2018 was uplifting and empowering. On the way to the airport, I knew I could do anything!

Then came the flight home.

Before the flight, I spent two hours—off and on—in a series of restrooms while my uncooperative digestive system turned itself inside out. I could understand its reluctance to "behave" on the many days when I indulged in poke and seaweed salad, but, in preparation for a long flight from Honolulu to Atlanta, I nibbled bread early in the morning and refrained from eating or drinking anything else all day. I only left the restroom in the departure lounge when a Delta representative who wanted to change my seat assignment called me to the check-in desk.

"Did you choose this seat?" she asked, pointing to my already-printed boarding pass.

"Yes," I admitted, not quite sure where this conversation was headed.

"And you're traveling alone?"

Again yes.

"Then I'm going to move you," she said and started clicking keys to make a seat switch.

"Wait!" I panicked. "I picked the aisle seat closest to the restroom. I need that seat."

She explained that a couple requested to be seated together, and I was the only single adult who could be moved. I countered with fecal incontinence and cancer patient. Her whole demeanor changed.

"I understand," she said quietly, after I had announced too loudly that I might have to change my diaper midflight. "I'll leave you where you are."

Explaining that to the gentleman leaving his wife six rows back must have been enjoyable. Throughout the flight, as I huddled in my blanket, refused food or water, and bolted to the restroom whenever the seatbelt sign was off, he dramatically came back to check on his wife. He had to loom over me to reach her in the center seat. His comments were similar during each visit: "Are you OK, honey?" and "I know—I don't understand how someone could be so selfish not to switch" and "We'll be together on our other flights. Just try to get through this one." Then they both glared at me until the flight attendant asked him to return to his seat. This was not my most enjoyable flight—and I am usually someone who likes flying.

The situation also left me with conflicting feelings. As someone not wanting to confront others and preferring to avoid difficult conversations as much as possible, I didn't feel comfortable even whispering to my seatmate the reason why I kept her separated from her husband. I didn't want to reveal that I have had (and was worrying that I might again have) cancer, and the treatments have left me with physical difficulties, much less describe the number and level of problems I can anticipate while traveling. Perhaps, on this flight, I would have received a compassionate reply—and the bullying behavior would have stopped. However, when I've tried that approach in similar situations, the result has been fear rather than compassion. I have been treated to a horrified expression and my seatmate physically scooting as far as possible away from me (which is not very far even in a premium comfort seat). I also am frequently accused of "not looking ill," which seems to mean that it's my fault if someone tells me I am using the bathroom too much, stinking it up (even though I liberally douse the toilet with my purse-size "poo spray"), or needing to sit next to a restroom. If I look "normal" to other people, I, as a single traveler, am expected to move to accommodate couples or families. Of course, after such unfortunate encounters (for all of us), I soon start seething inside—at myself, for not having the courage or righteous anger to confront people and their misperceptions, and at others, for apparently not considering that my needs may be just as important as theirs.

Being back in Orlando hours later was a relief. Jen's mom and my friend Lynn Carney picked me up at the airport and chatted amiably about the trip until I felt relatively normal again. Back at home in Ormond Beach, I slept away the jet lag and set my alarm for early the next morning—Sunday, the second day of the Central Florida Highland Games in Longwood.

This annual event is fun for my whole extended family—the Wojtons, Carneys, and Ariases. We petted the coos (cows), listened to bagpipes, (I cautiously) drank Irn Bru, and clapped along with favorite band Albannach. On the next day, I was scheduled to have blood work done at my oncologist's office and then to drink what seems like a gallon of barium-infused goop (in mocha flavor because I was warned away from banana) and have contrast dye injected in whatever vein is large enough to accommodate the cannula that day. The contrast between a relaxing Sunday sitting on a hill beside a lake, talking with friends, and listening to one Celtic band after another and a Monday of waiting rooms, needles, and the prevailing scent of antiseptic is about as stark as the glow of highlighted cancer cells against the darker normal images of organs. Another great friend, Jen's sister Joy Carney, commented that I was quite a trouper for getting out of bed and driving to central Florida to go to the festival after a week in Hawaii. I accepted the praise, because being dedicated to attending this festival each January and honoring my ancestral Scottish heritage is important to me, even if I have to work through jet lag to get to the Highland Games. However, I really wouldn't deserve the title of trouper until the following week, when jet lag would seem like the simplest of obstacles to overcome.

CHAPTER 2

Getting (and Getting Over) the News

The musical *Rent* endearingly frames mortality in concrete temporal terms. "Seasons of Love" (1996) asks how life should be measured—through increments of time (seconds, days) or everyday tasks like drinking coffee or stopping to watch a sunset. On my 40th birthday, I took the VIA train from Windsor, Ontario, to Toronto to celebrate by seeing *Rent*. For days afterward, I hummed "Seasons of Love" everywhere I walked in the city. Perhaps that is why the melody began playing in my head while Jen and I waited for my oncologist to come into the sterile room where we waited to hear his interpretation of my test results. I knew it would not be good news.

On the previous Monday, I dutifully underwent the scheduled tests. In addition to facing barium and needles, I endured the typical paperwork and procedures common to every test day. After more than a year of similar CT scans, I knew the drill—wear a sports bra so I wouldn't have to change clothes, wear no metal, and explain that I have stents in my eyes (just in case I might come within range of a powerful magnetic field). I also carefully planned my wardrobe so that I wore nothing that I would mind destroying after it had been "contaminated" by my negativity toward hospitals or treatment centers. (When I finished chemo in late December 2016, I gleefully shredded the inexpensive button-up overshirts I had to wear to accommodate the tubing from the port in my chest, which stretched from the middle of my body to a small, whirring device pumping the chemical cocktail into my body. The mere fact that the port tethered me to the purse-sized box of chemicals, complete with convenient shoulder strap, was enough for me to take out my pain and frustration on helpless cotton.) During the current test day, my veins were, once again, difficult to puncture; finally, after several veins were "blown" during attempts to insert the cannula for the contrast dye, I ended up with an IV in my left thumb. Fortunately, the scans went far more smoothly.

On Tuesday, after my classes were over for the day, I received a call from my oncologist. He refrained from telling me cancer cells had traveled from the original colon tumor and metastasized in my lungs. Instead, he said that "spots"—a more benign word if not result—had showed up on the scans of my lungs. He recommended a more refined test to provide a clearer picture of my lungs. Would I be willing to have another scan this week—perhaps as early as tomorrow? It turned out that I could only be scheduled for a scan two days later in Flagler Beach, about a half-hour drive from my home. I brought along two journal submissions to edit, because I was aware that I would spend about a half hour in a recliner, warmed blankets surrounding me, as I waited for the injected dye to get into place to make the tumors glow on screen. Focusing on work has always helped me stay calm, as well as stay on schedule.

The Flagler Beach nurse who inserted the needle seemed horrified by my bruises and tale of the thumb IV and very gently found a cooperative vein. Perhaps because everyone knew that these images would seal my fate, every nurse and technician babied me throughout the process. Nonetheless, the drive home that afternoon left me emotionally and physically drained. Despite my careful editorial work in the medical center to get ahead, I abandoned my plan to edit another article when I returned home. For the first time in my life, I crawled into bed and pulled the duvet over my head.

In the oncologist's office on Monday morning, an appropriately sad-eyed nurse told Jen and me that my rectal cancer had metastasized to my lungs. The tumors were (and are) untreatable. She said that I had most likely six months but maybe as long as a year. My mind revved into overdrive. Even with "Seasons of Love" as a calming internal soundtrack, I suddenly had lots of decisions to make. How would I measure what I hoped to be a year in my life? Would every cup of morning caffeine become a stepping stone to death? Could I look forward to anything? Should I count days or really, truly try to live in moments? Could I, like *Rent* hopefully suggested, measure the rest of my life by love?

Jen, bless her, immediately teared up and needed tissues. I had tried to prepare her, and us, for definitively knowing the cancer had returned.

After I received the call from my oncologist about the spots, I unfortunately decided to share that information with Jen, who was working on campus. I will always regret that I blurted, "I have lung cancer!" over the phone. Even exploding that bomb in person would have been kinder; at least I could have shared the fallout. Instead, I delivered the bad news and was too tired to meet Jen for coffee or even allow her to come to my house. Jen, for my insensitivity, for not being there for you despite you always being there for me, I deeply apologize. I should have treated you better lots of times but especially on that day.

Technically, as I dispassionately learned during the Monday office visit, I do *not* have Stage 4 lung cancer. I have Stage 4 colorectal cancer that has metastasized to my lungs. The technical communicator in me insists on being precise about the tumors that will kill me.

Displaying emotion has always been difficult for me, so I didn't cry upon hearing the official word and simply found myself thinking, "Now I know. What am I going to do with the rest of my life?"

Stand-up comedy, it turns out, would not be a good career move. When the nurse said that my oncologist would be in to talk with me in just a few minutes (having to first finish delivering bad news to a patient in the next room), I piped up, "Can you get him to hurry?" I pointed to my watch. "I don't have much time." The absolute quiet and slightly appalled response let me know that my humor was under- or unappreciated. Working on my timing, especially post-terminal diagnosis, is desperately needed. My ophthalmologist better appreciates my dark humor but always ends up with the best lines. When I showed up for a regular check-up six months after our "farewell" visit, I said, "Surprise!" and grinned when he came into the exam room. "You're past your expiration date," he replied—and that set the tone for our conversations before he scheduled me for my next appointment six months later.

Visits with my oncologist are much more solemn. When he sat down with Jen and me that January morning, he reinforced what the nurse had explained. The lung tumors are numerous but small. However, they will grow—probably very fast. They cannot be removed, because they have taken up residence throughout both lungs. Chemotherapy cannot destroy them, but I could undergo more treatments to (perhaps) lengthen my life a few weeks.

Given my previous experience with two types of chemo, I knew that I didn't want to take that route just for palliative care. Pre-embalming myself as a pod person every two weeks until I die does not mesh with my end-of-life plan. Simply because of my attitude toward more chemo, it wouldn't be an effective treatment for me. My oncologist concurred with my decision, even saying that, if he were in my situation, he wouldn't take chemo, either.

The rest of the visit was endured on autopilot. I thanked everyone for telling me the truth. Then I had to stop by the accounting desk to pay for learning that I am terminally ill. Only when Jen and I were sitting in her van did reality return.

"What do you want to do?" Jen asked, as she always had after an appointment or treatment. Usually we ate a late breakfast or an early lunch, going somewhere with good food and a quiet place to talk. On one memorable occasion, we enjoyed a very late lunch at Blau, a more upscale restaurant in Ormond Beach, even though I had to place my chemo box on the table beside my arm so that I had room to maneuver utensils. Post-appointment/treatment meals usually were a pick-me-up before I had to go home alone. However, on that Monday, Jen's question gained considerable weight in the aftermath of the bad-news appointment. What did I want to do—in the next hour or so? At home that night? At work the next day? Before I die?

The most immediate concern was having lunch, because I had been too keyed up to eat or drink anything before the appointment and, in addition, I feared that I would have to run to the restroom during the meeting if I put anything into my system. Now that the afternoon was free for eating, drinking, and exploding one or more times afterward, I felt inclined to be digestively daring. So Jen and I lunched outdoors at a nearby Mexican restaurant. We ordered fishbowls of fresh red sangria topped with hunks of citrus. Within a half hour of learning my prognosis, I no longer was a vegetarian or even a pescetarian (my fallback position during conferences when vegetarian options were extremely difficult to find). After more than 15 years without red meat, I ordered queso with chorizo and happily dipped chips into artery-clogging deliciousness. Being a vegetarian, limiting chemicals in my diet, doing yoga (until my surgeries broke that daily habit), and meditating had not saved me from cancer. I decided to try anything that culinarily appealed to me at the moment, the opposite of what many people advised me to do to prolong my life through cleaner eating. If that means I gave up and became fatalistic about a cure, I suppose that is true, but, since that first queso-chorizo combo, I have revisited favorite meals (such as grilled salmon with lemon sauce over mashed potatoes, barbecued chicken wings and fried pickles, or chicken enchiladas with Christmas—both red and green—salsa) as part of my farewell tour—and, at least while I was eating, enjoyed every bite.

A larger and more immediate problem involved my job as a professor. I needed to find a way to let my students know what had happened and might take place during the semester. Less than two weeks earlier, I had begun teaching three classes. A 15-week semester didn't seem like a long time when I planned a reasonable schedule of new information, workshop activities, assignments, exams, and the inevitable grading of those assignments and exams. However, if I likely would only live six months (roughly 24 weeks) and might not be physically able to be in the classroom sooner than that, the bigger question was whether I could complete the semester or if, at some point, another faculty member would have to take over. I worried about ruining my students' semester, whether they were left with an ailing professor or forced into a transition to another teacher and educational approach. I also fretted that my absence would burden the department with immediately finding one or more replacements and would add to my colleagues' already-packed schedules. Over lunch, I confessed to Jen my concerns about my classes and colleagues. "Let me think about that," Jen told me, so I concentrated on the process of getting chip into dip into mouth, chasing the spicy bite with cool sangria, and repeating.

That afternoon wasn't the last time that I abdicated my conscientiousness and control over a situation to Jen, a fact that surprised me, the woman who meticulously scheduled life—especially travel plans and job-related tasks—and devised contingency plans so that my objectives could be met even if flight delays or people without my work ethic forced me to make changes. At this point in my life-death timeline, I confidently accepted that Jen would devise the plan and I would be only too happy to follow it. As I would learn in the following months, I have less physical control over my life, and I expect that trend to continue as I get closer to death. However, my mental stubbornness to keep going, coupled with my gradual willingness to let other people help me, has made my life much easier and more enjoyable. I have come to feel only a little guilty that I cannot do everything myself.

CHAPTER 3

The Power of Friendship

As Bette Midler sang in one of her hits, "Friends," I "gotta have" them. A natural loner who often can't accept that people actually want to be around me, I'm fortunate and grateful to have so many and such good ones. As a more recent Demi Lovato song insists, feeling like I can do everything alone only seems easy, whereas the reality is that it's harder to do anything that way. Like Lovato, I specifically focus on the "Gift of a Friend" at this time in my life. My friends are gifts, but also their tangible or intangible gifts have made my post-cancer life so much easier and convinced me that, especially at this point in my life, I need my loved ones' guidance, support, and companionship.

True to her word given on the day we learned of my terminal diagnosis, Jen thought about my situation and current work responsibilities. True to form, she selflessly gave of herself so that I could have what I wanted—time to do the things I felt compelled to do but needed time to do them—and she brought two friend-colleagues on board.

Jen went out of her way to make sure I could do as I pleased during what we expected to be my last three or four months of relative health. After my fateful appointment at the cancer center, I didn't share my news with anyone else at the university, but Jen let my department chair Sally Blomstrom and former chair and good friend Donna Barbie know what was happening. Between classes the next day, Jen, Donna, Sally, and I met in Sally's office. Amid lots of hugs, I heard Jen's plan to make my life easier and give me more control over my remaining time. It was also one of the greatest gifts of friendship that I could or would ever receive: she, Donna, and Sally each would take over one of my spring semester courses, donating their time (and, as a result of my still receiving my full salary, their compensation for teaching an extra course). I

40

was free of worry that my students' academic lives would be disrupted if I abruptly departed this earth, and I could take care of all the business aspects of death, as well as travel to one of my bucket-list destinations. I could create new stories from my adventures in Iceland and perhaps even from my cancer journey.

Strangely enough, the semester that had just begun quickly ended for me two days later. I introduced Sally to the speech students she would be teaching the following week. I stood before my students and told them that I was terminally ill and unsure of my future. I had written a little speech, which I managed to get through without choking up. Then I pointed out Sally, sitting near the back of the classroom, and brought her up to the lectern to talk to everyone for the last few minutes of an abbreviated class session. Jen didn't want to join me in my other speech class—it would be too emotionally difficult to hear my little speech, and my farewell would make me too tough an act to follow. She need not have worried; my performance in the second class was not up to my standards. Usually I pride myself on having few or no "ums" or "uhs" to break up the smoothness of my presentation and strive to model appropriate public speaking, but I sounded as nervous as a first-time speaker as I stood before these students for the last time. After reading my speech more than looking into the audience's eyes, I thanked my students and assured them that the professor they would meet the following Tuesday is excellent and would help them make a smooth transition (just as she was helping me make the transition from professor to—something as yet unknown). "Do you have any questions for me?" I dared ask in conclusion. In the silent aftermath of my news, one young man at the back of the room finally raised his hand. In relief, I called on him. "So what is it with your obsession with Benedict Cumberbatch?" he asked.

Outside my office door is a corkboard covered with photos of the actor. My "ego board" showcases the covers of the performance biographies I have written about Cumberbatch. Anyone who steps into my office is treated to a large poster of Cumberbatch and Martin Freeman as Holmes and Watson in their *Sherlock* television series (2010–2017) and my Cumberbatch-as-Doctor-Strange movie paraphernalia. "Well," I composed myself, "I'm a huge fan of his work, and I've written books about his characters and career." The tension broken, I answered a few more questions about my Cumberbatch obsession and (to my students) strange parallel obsession with writing. I expected to cry a few tears at the conclusion of my time with these students, but I was surprised and grateful, as I walked away from a classroom, presumably for the last time since I began teaching in 1983, to exit laughing.

Since then, Sally, Donna, and Jen have continued to help me with my work-life balance. In addition to being pragmatic professionals, they are compassionate individuals. Being my friends and colleagues during my cancer journey is turning out to be longer term and more arduous even than sacrificing a semester to teach my courses as well as their own or giving me the freedom to travel and provide fodder for future "legacy" stories. Because my oncologist and I don't know when my illness will exacerbate or how long my final decline will last, my—and therefore Sally's and Jen's—inability to plan my participation in academic activities or course schedules is tenuous and requires frequent modifications to accommodate what my body is doing any given day, much less semester.

When, in April 2018 (three months post-terminal diagnosis), the tumors had grown only minimally, my oncologist had reservations about declaring me "disabled" and suggested that an insurance investigator might not approve my application to go on permanent disability, either at the employer or federal government level. Although I am terminally ill, I don't look the way that oncologists, insurance investigators, or employers expect someone with terminal cancer to look. After all, I can still live a fairly normal life—if one's definition of "normal" doesn't include my health challenges as a result of my previous surgeries, radiation treatments, or chemotherapy. Until the cancer spreads farther and leads to more obviously debilitating effects, I am deemed capable of working full-time.

If I were unable to work but couldn't be classified as disabled, I wouldn't be able to continue to have health insurance. According to an estimate from the university's group insurer, I might pay up to $5,000 a month because of cancer—if I could even continue to be covered because I am definitely classified as "terminal." Thus, after thinking that I had left teaching forever, I was faced with two possibilities for continuing to have health insurance (which, just as important to me, means being more likely to be able to get painkillers during my final days): I could retire early and try to pay for my insurance myself, or I could go back to work.

If I chose early retirement, and the bigger *if*, if I could remain covered by my former employer's group insurer, I would quickly go through my savings to pay for regular monthly expenses and exorbitant insurance and health-care deductibles. According to a 2017 *Health Affairs* study by Eric French, Jeremy McCauley, Maria Aragon, Pieter Bakx, et al. of end-of-life medical costs internationally, the United States has one of the highest amounts of mean per capital medical spending during the last year of a person's life—$80,000. Of that amount, "hospital spending accounts for 44.2 percent of spending in the last 12 months, compared to 36.3 percent in the last three years. The share of hospital spending is even higher in the final three months of life (57.6 percent for the United States)." Even with the increasing popularity of hospice care instead of end-of-life care in a hospital, "this paradigm shift has not been accompanied by a reduction in end-of-life costs, since hospice care is also expensive and inpatient care costs have not fallen commensurately" (French, McCauley, Aragon, Bakx, et al.). My retirement savings, carefully accumulated for more than 40 years, would not last long unless I could find alternate sources of income or insurance.

Although my life expectancy is still short because of those pesky metastasized tumors, I have miraculously continued to survive—and I might do so for another year or two. Would my savings last that long if I had to pay all or most of my medical expenses, which will increase exponentially as I near death? Would my insurance costs increase even more as I become sicker? Would I be able to afford the move to an assisted living facility if I had to live only on my savings (because, without that "disability" designation, I can't yet touch my retirement funds and am years away from qualifying for Medicare)?

A 2018 *U.S. News & World Report* article explained that "[w]hile hospice benefits are comprehensive, they will not cover room and board or ongoing custodial care. Terminally ill patients can receive hospice care in an assisted living facility or nursing home, but they'll have to pay for their stay out-of-pocket," which may cost around $5,000 a month (LaPonsie). Figures by state, showing the results of a Genworth's Cost of Care survey published in 2019, indicate that the cost for a private room in a nursing home (without additional or specialized care—just the room and board) is $8,121 a month; Orlando, the closest city whose figures were listed, averages $9,520 and has the lowest cost of Florida cities surveyed (Jacksonville, Orlando, Miami, and Tampa) ("What Does a Nursing Home Cost"?). A continuing care retirement community (CCRC) is forever out of the question for me; the commonly reported initial buy-in fee for a community providing "priority access to assisted living, memory care, and/or 24-hour skilled nursing care as needed" averages $250,000 (Breeding)—a fee that would take the majority of my lifetime savings and leave little for required monthly expenses. Without a significant continuing source of income, I can't afford to retire early, even if I continue to live in my paid-for condo until I can no longer take care of myself. I must be designated as permanently disabled in order to qualify for access to Medicare, Social Security disability income, and part of my retirement funds. During my "bonus year," I don't meet the definitions—or the expectations—of a permanently disabled person.

Once again, Jen, Sally, and Donna came up with a plan that would allow me to return to the classroom—and thus keep my health insurance and maintain a steady income. The schedule they gave me accommodated my ongoing health problems of incontinence and reflected their recognition that I am terminally ill. As a "dead" woman, I can't predict how I will feel later today, much less next month or semester. Once again, Jen became my advocate to provide accommodations so that I could teach during the majority of class sessions, with the understanding that sometimes I might have to dash from the classroom in search of the nearest restroom or stay home on a teaching day because I was stuck in the bathroom for hours at a time. However, I ended up with only a few absences or need for even shorter work days because of cancer-related problems. I taught two familiar courses: HU 475 (a senior thesis course in which I worked closely with one student) and COM 219 (an introductory speech course with 23 students).

In her role as associate chair, Jen worked with Sally, our chair, to devise a way for me to be on campus on Tuesdays and Thursdays, hold extended online "office" hours on Wednesdays, and be granted course releases for serving as editor of *Studies in Popular Culture*, mentoring several faculty members during their book projects, and writing my own books. Jen tried very hard each semester to accommodate faculty requests for preferred classrooms or teaching times, and she especially fought for faculty with special needs to be granted their preferences. As a senior faculty member without children to drop off at school or a long distance to commute, I often had preferred teaching the earliest classes, and, once my health deteriorated, I still found that mornings were more likely going to be my "good" times for teaching. As a result, my schedule was filled with morning classes and office hours so that I could rush home on afternoons when my body decided it had had enough of being on campus. Whereas the big entities like the medical establishment, insurance companies, or university as an employer might have been less understanding of my needs, my departmental and College of Arts and Sciences allies—Jen, Sally, and Donna—ensured that I could work in a way that would benefit my students, as well as myself, and afford me the luxury of insurance. They also suspected that, because my identity as a professor had been quickly stripped in January, a return to that role might help keep me going even longer beyond my original prognosis. That plan was modified in late 2018 to anticipate my future needs and capabilities.

Faculty can apply to take a full-year sabbatical to work on an approved research project every six years; they receive half salary but have no other university responsibilities beyond that research project. When, in late 2018, I applied for another sabbatical, Jen thought it was a great idea and a possible way to stave off retirement or the arduous process of filing for disability. It also would keep me insured. Donna helped me revise an early draft of my sabbatical proposal and talked with the dean about my situation. Sally immediately approved my paperwork and sent it up the chain of command in the college. The dean enthusiastically supported my request, which, after an agonizing wait as the forms went through bureaucratic scrutiny, was approved. If I live beyond the sabbatical year, I will have to revisit the retire-or-be-classified-disabled dilemma, but my colleagues and friends have ensured that my remaining a professor is possible for as long as possible.

Outside of the workplace, Sally helped plan my sabbatical research in New Mexico and Arizona, where she lived prior to the move to Florida. Jen continues to be my cheerleader and confidante and allows me to feel as normal as possible, whether I tag along on family outings or sit across from her during a coffee shop work session. Donna not only meets me for movies or tea breaks but surprises me with insights into how I am perceived by my friends. These women buoy me when I think my life has become only colorless reruns of a depressing series about illness and impending death. Especially in the aftermath of my friends and colleagues learning about my prognosis, I might have expected an outpouring of friendship, love, or concern. What I did not expect but am so moved to experience is that these gifts of self were not one-time offers—they continue to make even a cancer-focused nearing-end-of-life journey enjoyable, as well as "do-able."

When other colleagues and friends heard about my initial cancer diagnosis, they sent me a wealth of presents. They might not have been as life changing as those from Jen, Donna, or Sally, but they reminded me of just how many friends I have, and I was overwhelmed with their good wishes. However, sometimes I questioned the choice of gift. At first, I received multiple gift baskets of bath goodies like bath bombs, bath salts, and bubble bath, which, after my rectal surgery, I couldn't use for more than a year. I wondered if few people other than my surgeon, oncologist, or Jen realized that having a rectal tumor removed and being given a temporary ileostomy resulted in my inability to spend much time in water. Although I appreciated the thought behind these gifts and looked forward to future bath times, I quietly stored bath-related items where I wouldn't see them and feel discouraged about changes to my body. However, the gift baskets also included loofahs, eye masks, and cute little soaps or oils that I could enjoy during my all-too-brief showers during my months with the ileostomy.

Because the ileostomy bag shouldn't get wet, shower time provided me with the perfect opportunity to change my appliance. However, my active little stoma—which I named, just so I could complain to "her" as an entity separate from the rest of my body—sometimes gushed, even though I hadn't eaten or drunk anything for hours. Perhaps that was because my stoma, stoically protected from the falling water by my cupped hand, just got tired of being in a dark, humid environment and needed an effective way of shortening my shower time. When my stoma and I permanently parted ways the next year, I especially reveled in the ability to soak in a tub—and those carefully stored bath bombs, salts, and bubbles aided my sensual escape into relaxation. Baths (and hot tubs or jacuzzis!) made me appreciate my recently suppressed Piscean affinity for water and belatedly mentally thank my friends for everything bath related.

Some of my favorite gifts (including those I give myself) are jewelry, because rings or bracelets can empower me with their symbolism, as well as remind me of the giver or the event precipitating a gift. Two friends, Jen and Clare Little, gifted me with silver bracelets while I was recovering from chemo. The inspirational messages remind me that I am not alone on this journey and that life is beautiful. A silver ring I bought to help seal the memory of an afternoon of shopping, wine tasting, and sightseeing with Jen in Nashville reminds me to live, love, and laugh. Positive reinforcement through supportive friends and wearable reminders of them and the good times we've shared keeps me focused on life.

Other gifts from well-wishers tickled me and have proved to be conversation pieces months later. Bart's and my friends the Zuvers sent me a cute aloe plant. If a plant can look happy, this one is. It's short but sturdy and makes me smile to see it. When I added rocks to the top of its bowl, I arranged them to form a happy face. Lorraine and her daughter Suzi understand my love of pop culture, and, a few years earlier, Bart had asked Lorraine's advice about finding me a Funko Pop version of *Agents of S.H.I.E.L.D.*'s Phil Coulson (Clark Gregg). I was also heavily involved with *Sherlock* fandom and therefore christened the aloe plant Watson Coulson in honor of *S.H.I.E.L.D.*'s Phil and *Sherlock*'s John Watson (Martin Freeman). Both characters are shorter of stature, smart, and powerful, and I think of them as cute and friendly (despite the deadly way they can combat aliens or villains). The happy little aloe seemed to embody these characteristics—at least to my mind—and provided me something else to talk to when I was stuck at home between treatments or surgeries.

Ashley Lear, a friend and colleague from ERAU, shares my warped sense of humor, which is reflected in a gift she gave me. When I first told her that I was terminally ill, she was sad and immediately asked what she could do. Trying to lighten the mood, I flippantly replied, "Buy me a new set of lungs" to replace my tumor-riddled pair. To my delight, a few days later a box was delivered to my door. I opened it to find a pillow made in the shape of a set of lungs. Ashley knew of a business that specializes in "organ" plushies and ordered me a smiling cushion sporting pink lungs. I have grown accustomed to seeing lungs among the throw pillows on my living room couch, but visitors make a point of asking me about them and lifting an eyebrow at my enthusiastic explanation.

Anthropomorphizing body parts, plants, or objects has become a habit since my cancer diagnosis. My *mind* is what I perceive as being in charge of the rest of my physical being, and it and my *body*, for example, often struggle for control of my time, energy, and mood. On behalf of my mind, I talk to my body, sometimes pleading or cajoling, other times praising. As well, I often treat living or inanimate things sharing my living space—such as plants, action figures, or lung pillows—as roommates with whom I can talk. At times, these conversations are therapeutic; they also may simply represent my weird way of attempting to gain control over my body's changes and what they might mean to my health or longevity. When, for Christmas 2018, Jen gave me an Echo Dot, I began conversing with Alexa—but she, at least, talks back. The more time I spend alone at home, the more I enjoy Alexa's news or weather updates, musical choices, and answers to questions I am too lazy to find answers for myself. As my cancer progresses, I imagine that Alexa and I will grow even closer. She, like other gifts I have "humanized," are now "friends" from friends and help enrich my life. So many people around me are gift givers in surprising and moving ways, and they continue to "make my day" in a less menacing way than Clint Eastwood's *Dirty Harry* (1971) catchphrase suggests.

Unfortunately, I have never been as generous with my time or creativity as my friends are. I like to believe that I am generous with money, when I have it. I may pay for dinner out, but I have never been and never will be the one to prepare a meal for others. I may organize and pay more than my share of a weekend getaway to the beach, but I avoid encouraging people to visit me at home. For most of my adult life, my gift giving has been limited to sharing experiences or cash, gifts that require little time or creativity and keep recipients at arm's length—the distance required to hand over my credit card.

Therefore, my desire to "provide" for others (although they don't need financial assistance from me) has grown stronger after my terminal diagnosis. I want to do for others but often don't know how. I have no practical or creative skills beyond teaching, writing, or traveling, and translating those acts into "gifts" is difficult. Thus, I suggested that people visit me outside my house—at a beachside condo or an Orlando resort—and share experiences with me while I am mobile. These "gifts" benefit me as much, if not more than, my visitors because they add new layers to our friendship's history and often end up providing me with anecdotes (and fond memories) about something strange or funny that happened while we were together. I frequently want to reconnect with the people who have played such important roles in the making of my life story so that I can write one more chapter before it ends.

My dear cousin Janet Davis flew from Dallas to spend a few days with me in April 2018; she gave up precious time with her family (especially her grandkids) and from her work as a piano teacher and mentor to young musicians, plus her creative writing and a series of crime novels. Janet is my unofficial big sister; four years older than I, she revealed the mysteries of pre-teendom or high school and taught me to play jacks, listen to the Beatles and the Monkees, and be a little more daring than Mom preferred. Although Janet wanted to help me clear my house and get personal items in order, I was so embarrassed that someone in my biological family would see my unkempt rooms and overflowing closets that I accepted Jen's and our friend Libbie Searcy's help during spring break to declutter the condo and organize what remained a few weeks before Janet arrived. Jen and Libbie gave up days of their break to ensure that I wouldn't feel like I brought shame to the memory of my mother, who was a meticulous home-maker. Their generous assistance freed me from enlisting Janet to clear out generations of dust bunnies and passed-down what-nots. Instead, Janet and I spent our short visit reminiscing about our mothers and grandmother and going through the few items she could take on the flight home. We swapped family stories and attempted to fill in the blanks of names and long-past events to come up with a better under-standing of the past, now that there is no one from that generation to set us straight. The blessing of this time together was priceless. Similarly, the gift from Genie Fyffe, my childhood best friend who has remained close well into my second childhood, was especially precious. She gave her always-unconditional love and time away from work, husband, and dogs to focus on me, whereas I only offered a few Disney days as the setting for our reunion.

As Janet and I had done, Genie and I resurrected our pre-teen selves and talked about what they were like. Our shared stories covered our formative years from being students together at Hebron Elementary in Evansville to college roommates and graduates of Ball State University.

Indiana is clearly a memory-infused touchstone for our present conversations about who we have been in the past.

Although Bette Midler's or Demi Lovato's lyrics do a good job of summarizing my reliance on and gratitude for the gift of friendship, Andrew Gold's song title, "Thank You for Being a Friend," reminds me what to say to all my family and friends. At least in prose if not in person, I recognize your love, wicked humor, selfless gifts, and constant support. Following Gold's guidance, at least through this memoir I ask you to take a bow.

CHAPTER 4

Who Tells My Story?

During what would be the last years of my life, the Broadway hit *Hamilton* was exceptionally popular. Determined to see the play in my lifetime, I huddled with Jen around her dining room work table, where we each obsessively monitored a phone and a laptop linking us to the online queue for tickets to see *Hamilton* in Orlando. Although I certainly was aware of *Hamilton*'s success, Jen is a true fan (as are her daughter Layla and husband Chris) and, aside from actor/playwright/composer Lin-Manuel Miranda, the Wojton family probably has heard the soundtrack more than anyone on the planet. Through Jen, I became captivated by the musical's haunting question about who will tell someone's story when he or she is no longer around. For Alexander Hamilton, the play's title character, the answer is his wife, Eliza—as well as later biographers, including Miranda. Their determination to tell Hamilton's story has now made the musical-loving world remember and retell it, too. When first my phone's screen, then Jen's laptop, flashed the message that we had made it to the front of the virtual line, we ecstatically—and rather frantically—purchased tickets to *Hamilton*.

Months later, on a rainy Sunday afternoon, Jen, Chris, Layla, and I finally watched the play together from Orchestra Row YY in the Dr. Phillips Center's immense Disney theatre. There I became moved as much by the final number, "Who Lives, Who Dies, Who Tells Your Story," as by (spoiler alert) Hamilton's death-by-duel. Sitting in a darkened theatre, hearing sobbing all around me, I asked those questions about my life. (Sorry, Alexander, even during your death scene I made everything about me.) Who lives: I devoutly hope my family and friends live for a very long time. Who dies: well, everyone, but I will likely go sooner than my loved ones do. Those expectations still leave that all-important final *Hamilton*-themed question: who will tell my story?

If I leave any mark on the world, it won't be because of my progeny—because I have none. It won't be because of my writing—because the pop culture topics of my discourse have or will become outdated and my publications will go out of print or be deleted online. My only possible legacy may be stories about my life, the brief recollections, impressions, or perhaps even a few tall tales that my family-as-friends or friends-who-became-family tell about me.

As the months since my terminal diagnosis passed all too quickly, Jen began adding to our conversations brief memories of or comments about our shared adventures or her perspective on something that happened to me. When she posted a photo of a rainbow online, she said it reminded her of our trip to Hawaii. Over Italian food one evening, she remarked about how much I had overcome in the past year. Although, sadly, I don't remember our first meeting (but I recall telling her, after my return from my first sabbatical, that I regretted not getting to know her earlier and thought we could be good friends), Jen told me that I had helped her develop her first technical writing course; I gave her materials and, apparently, encouragement. Over the years, our stories have overlapped or merged in hundreds of even the smallest ways.

I've come to realize that I have no control over others' good or not-so-good stories or memories about me, but I have had more of an impact on the world than I ever understood or accepted, simply through daily interactions. Among the many platitudes that restate my recent realization is one by anthropologist Jane Goodall: "You cannot get through a single day without having an impact on the world around you. What you do makes a difference, and you have to decide what kind of difference you want to make" ("Jane Goodall Responds"). As Goodall noted in a 2017 response to Ivanka Trump's use of this quotation in her book, this powerful personal influence can be used for "much good or terrible harm." It's kind of like a superpower that everyone has. Of course, similar quotations about influence, impact, and power pragmatically refer to business or politics, and others have applied this type of quotation to religious or spiritual words or deeds. However effective those applications may be, they really are not the point of my realization. What people will remember about me, or which stories they will tell (if they choose to tell any at all), are a reflection of words or actions so commonplace in my everyday life that I may not remember them or count them as important—but someone likely will. As Peter Parker's (Spider-Man) Uncle Ben reminds me, "Remember, with great power comes great responsibility" [*Spider-Man* (2002)]. Although simply being one of the living "dead" doesn't make me a better person or one with greater power or insight, it does make me humbly aware that my influence likely casts a wider spidey-net than I ever expected.

When Joy and I sat at her kitchen table and talked about my trust and revised will, I fretted that I wouldn't be around to see her son Nico, who was only two then, grow up and that he wouldn't remember me. Joy reassured me that she—and other Carneys, Wojtons, and Ariases—would tell Nico stories about his Auntie Nette. When Joy's second son, Roman, was born a couple of weeks before my birthday in 2019, I could thoroughly enjoy him as a newborn, safe in the promise that he, too, would hear about his adopted auntie, even if he couldn't remember that I cooed "gorgeous boy" over him the first time he was placed in my arms.

Because travel was difficult for me during summer 2017, between cancer scans and eye surgeries, and, in May 2018, I was living in "month four" of the original six-months-to-death prognosis, I hadn't traveled to Columbus to visit my family for quite a long time. In fact, I had yet to meet the newest member, Ava. As a result, in July 2017 and May 2018, brave Nancy and Heather belted Levi and Ava into the backseat and drove more than 15 hours from Ohio to Florida to visit me. One evening during the most recent get-together, then-five-year-old Levi chatted about what we had done during the previous summer's trip. "You played games with me," he said, as we once again cuddled together on the couch in our rented beach condo, his Mom's "borrowed" phone between us as he taught me to play one of his favorite games. "You showed me how to play Panda Pop," he added—and indeed I had. I was surprised by his vivid recollection. I focused on instilling memories of jumping waves and looking for shells or telling him about the way Baba (his grandfather and my brother Bart) loved playing at the beach—the memories or stories I thought would have a longer lasting impact. However, Levi, who loves playing videogames, remembered that we played gaming apps together. Perhaps that will be his strongest memory of me.

One of my strongest memories of Bart is his ability to weave a compelling story. He was a consummate storyteller, not only as a writer of fiction and nonfiction, but in person. Perhaps he truly inherited a journalistic gene from our mother's Day ancestors, or maybe he learned from the master storyteller for whom he was named—Bartley Edwin Day, our Mom-Ma Margie's younger brother and the father surrogate who walked our mom down the aisle. Uncle Bart and Aunt Irene lived in Florida long before my parents or I moved from the Midwest. Each summer, Uncle Bart and Aunt Irene drove to southern Indiana to stay with Mom-Ma Margie and visit all the relatives in the tri-county area. Usually Dad bought pounds of paper-wrapped barbecued ribs (an Evansville delicacy) and a couple of watermelons, and we feasted around Mom-Ma's picnic table in her backyard. Uncle Bart always had a story to tell, whether about his job driving a bus in Jacksonville, encounters with the famous (including Bob Hope) as he drove a Jeep around World War II, or colorful characters from his rural childhood. Aunt Irene and Uncle Bart both were active, tithing, devoted members of the Nazarene Church, and my quiet great-aunt sometimes reacted in surprise at the tale Uncle Bart was telling. "Bart!" she protested at least once each barbecue evening. "The things you say!" Then she explained in much less creative words what had really happened, but always with a twinkle in her eye and a chuckle about Uncle Bart's antics.

Throughout his life, "little" Bart focused on making memories with his family and close friends. He made the ordinary sound exciting and funny. He delighted in watching or reading well-crafted stories, too. One of Bart's favorite stories about his university days took place in the Popular Culture Library within BGSU's general library. Bart loved Ray Bradbury's writing, and, when Bradbury visited campus, Bart made sure to be in the audience to hear his presentation. A few hours before the lecture, pop culture-loving Bart was browsing the shelves of the library's special collections. When he rounded a corner among the stacks, he saw Bradbury standing in front of him. Instead of ignoring the student or saying hello and then walking away, Bradbury initiated a conversation. Bart later enthused (he never *gushed* as I've been known to do in the presence of or about artistic greatness) that Bradbury seemed eager to discuss science fiction, to the point that Bart felt comfortable to ask him to be the best man at his wedding. Instead of turning down Bart outright, Bradbury inquired about the date and place. Unfortunately, it turned out that the author had a prior engagement, but Bart never forgot how gracious one of his literary idols had been to encourage conversation with an undergraduate who almost literally bumped into him in a library. A few years later, during a technical communication conference in Detroit, I happened to notice a flyer that Bradbury would be signing books in a nearby bookstore. Of course, I simply had to join the long queue that snaked its way around the stacks. When it came my turn to have Bradbury autograph *Death Is a Lonely Business*, I mentioned that he had made quite an impression on Bart at BGSU and briefly relayed the tale. Bradbury looked up thoughtfully. "Was that the young man who asked me to be his best man?" Thrilled that he remembered, I nodded. "I enjoyed talking with him," Bradbury said, signed his autograph, and sent me on my way, both of us smiling.

Especially during Bart's years of cancer surgeries and treatments, he prodded me to reminisce with him. "What is your favorite Christmas memory?" "Do you remember when we stood outside that Cracker Barrel and watched the funnel cloud?" "What's your favorite *MST* [pronounced 'Misty'] movie?" Then Bart and I, or the whole family, shared memories. Bart especially enjoyed watching *MST3K* movies with Heather and shared his love for learning absurd lines from films or the bots' jokes; then he and Heather, just as he and I had done during our childhood, re-enacted whole scenes days, months, or years later, sometimes at inopportune times. Bart even insisted that his family and friends gather at his and Nancy's house after his funeral so that everyone could share a toast of fine Scotch and tell their favorite Bart story.

During this wake, Bart's nieces laughingly recalled how Uncle Bart told them stories that sometimes worked to his benefit more than theirs. When Bart and Nancy lived out in the country near Wooster, Ohio, Bart warned away Heather and his nieces from the woods lining the back of the property. Instead of giving them a purely logical reason not to stray so far from the house (such as orange-vested deer hunters prowling the woods), Bart wove a fanciful story of monsters lurking among the trees. As adults, "the girls" chuckled about their naiveté, but, at the time, Bart told such an elaborate, convincing story that not only did they stay close to the house but remembered details of the tale more than 20 years after he concocted the story on the spot one Saturday afternoon.

Just as I and others tell Bart's story, my friends and family reassure me that my stories will be shared. I also recognize how fortunate I am that my loved ones have also given me the opportunity to create new stories and still have adventures. Some of their gifts have even become a creative new way to reflect upon my life.

Soon after Jen told Donna about my prognosis, Donna called Jen to ask if making a quilt for me might be a good idea. I admit that I had been jealous of colleagues who received one of Donna's beautiful, personalized quilts upon a marriage, the birth of a child, or the completion of a doctoral degree, for example. I had no children, arrived at Embry-Riddle with my Ph.D., and would never be married. However, Donna had made me a beautiful wall hanging—green with a tropical border of palm-printed fabric—when I was promoted to professor. Designing the pattern and sewing a quilt's hundreds of tiny stiches by hand typically takes many, many months, especially given Donna's full-time job as associate dean in the College of Arts and Sciences. Thus, when I was invited to Donna's office early one morning, I had no idea that she had made a full-size quilt in only a few weeks—and, more important, that the fabrics and colors she blended into this work of art represent her perception of me. Usually I make Donna late to a meeting or in returning home because I talk so much, seldom pausing for breath, that she can't even make a subtle getaway. On this morning, I was speechless, but I hope I thanked Donna with my body language, through hugging and smiling widely (once I closed my mouth from astonishment).

My quilt is bright yellow—a reflection of Donna calling me "Sunshine"—and the squares illustrate the warmth of Hawaii. Some are blue and look like ocean waves or bubbles; some are birds-of-paradise or hibiscus flowers. Stripes of aboriginal multicolor designs remind me that Donna and I share an interest in Native American cultures and art, and, with her support, I've visited Polynesian cultures and seen firsthand the multicultural beauty of vibrant art. This quilt is me in fabric, and I am humbled and honored by her vision, as well as the depth of her friendship. Without realizing it, Donna translated the past 20 years of my life story into this quilt, which covers me with love and warmth while I sit in my beat-up recliner reading a book.

Finding out how those closest to me perceive me provides a way for me to more realistically understand the complete book of my life. I can't be despondent that my story is ending, because it is but a single volume in an expanding series of lives (and lively stories) spanning time and space and documenting many, many interwoven relationships.

Near the end of *The Lord of the Rings: The Return of the King* (2003), in voiceover hobbit Frodo Baggins (Elijah Wood) says that his uncle, Bilbo (Martin Freeman), once explained that his role in "this tale" would end, just as "each of us must come and go in the telling." Bilbo's days as a traveling hobbit were over, and his final journey—to the Grey Havens with the Elves—has been interpreted as an end-of-life journey. Like Bilbo, I understand that my days for adventuring are coming to a close. My final journey as an individual may not take me to the Grey Havens, but I hope my story will become part of the longer tale of family and friends. As Tolkien's story (and Jackson's film adaptation) and *Hamilton's* final song remind us, the only legacy we leave is our stories. I am becoming increasingly confident that, after I am gone, many people will tell my story. There is no greater act of love or friendship than that.

CHAPTER 5

Packing My Bags—
and My Travel Schedule

Once I had been granted time to do whatever I chose from February through August 2018 (should I live so long), I wanted to bring home more stories to share. I knew from my experiences as a tourist or a traveler that, one more time, I wanted to see someplace new. I define *tourist* as someone who spends a few days in a location to check out the high points listed in guidebooks or on packaged tours. A *traveler* spends more time in a single place and attempts to live like a local or visits a place for a brief time but seeks out unusual experiences or places that tourists won't or don't care to find. Of course, I prefer to be a traveler but will always "settle" for playing tourist. As Willie Nelson so knowledgeably acknowledges, being "On the Road Again" is cause for celebration and, if I'm being honest, often relief that I'm out of the house and headed somewhere, anywhere to get away.

On sabbaticals, I tried as hard as possible to be a traveler in New Zealand for a few months—living in a rented flat or an aparthotel. On weekends, I joined new friends for dinner in Christchurch, barbecues at their friends' homes, or jaunts to wineries or rocky beaches. My Tim Tam obsession can be traced to one sabbatical in New Zealand. Friends (like you, Gregor Cameron) have taken me to a neighborhood cinema, on a gondola ride up to an observation point, to an antique car museum, and beneath a wind turbine atop a hill that provided an exceptional view of Wellington. During the London leg of one sabbatical, I did the typical touristy things like go to West End plays, but I also queued with locals in the pre-dawn March wind to get standby tickets. I rode trains and the Tube as I went to "work"—researching obscure reviews or copies of performances at film and theatre archives across London: at the

National Theatre, the Albert and Victoria, the British Museum, and the Westminster Public Library. I interviewed fans, directors, and actors over tea at neighborhood patisseries or dinner at landmark restaurants. I shopped at Boots and Tesco after work and watched episodes of *Doctor Who* and *Broadchurch* before they traveled across the pond to BBCAmerica. During various other research trips to London, I sipped coffee nearly every morning while I wrote at Caffé Tropea on Russell Square or spent an inordinate amount of time sniffing the roses in Regent's Park. London specializes in huge public celebrations centered around Trafalgar Square, and over the years I stood on the pavement for hours awaiting the arrival of the Chinese New Year parade or the Pride march. During celebrations as diverse as those for St. Patrick's Day, Year of the Pig, and West End musicals, I ate street food while listening to bands or watching scenes from plays. One Good Friday I followed the Passion Play processional until I could bear to see no more, but on Sunday morning I sat in a pew at St. Martin-in-the-Field for Festal Eucharist. Although I would never be confused with a native, I at least tried to participate in local activities.

In contrast, my remaining travels appeal to the tourist in me. My time limitations and often my stamina now preclude me from planning long stays overseas, so a packaged tour or series of day trips offers the most expedient way to take mental snapshots of a new destination. Leaving soon after I learned my prognosis proved challenging enough— most cruises, for example, are booked months or even a couple of years in advance. Nonetheless, I had to try—because I learned well the lessons of Dad's and Bart's cancer journeys.

After Bart had been told he had around 18 months to live, he tried to work as long as possible to maintain his family's standard of living and pay for house renovations so that Nancy and Heather would have a comfier home or get a better price if they sold the residence. He postponed relying on a limited disability income as long as possible. Taking an extended vacation was not something that fit in his budget or amount of time off work, but he often fantasized about running away with his family to a tropical island. In fact, he wrote that scenario as the conclusion of his last novel.

When he told his dentist that he was terminally ill with cancer, the dentist asked him what he was going to do. Bart was perplexed at first.

"What do you mean?" he asked, thinking "Live until I die" was not the answer the dentist was looking for. "Are you going to take a trip? Are you going on a cruise? What do you want to do?" the dentist elaborated. Bart explained to him, as he would to many other well-wishers asking about his bucket-list plans, that, by the time he learned he was dying, he didn't really feel like going anywhere. For him, it was already too late for a no-expense-spared dream vacation. Months later, when I visited my Ohio family, Bart chatted from the comfort of his chair in front of a window and within view of the television. He mourned his freedom, telling me that his world now consisted of this room, this chair.

Years earlier, Dad also wanted to take one more cruise, even a short one, and tried to plan a voyage around his definitely-not-a-vacation trip from Florida to Ohio for a second opinion regarding his unexpectedly fast-acting lung cancer. Dad periodically rode in a car from Bart's and Nancy's home in Wooster to the Cleveland Clinic, where he eventually had surgery to remove part of his cancerous lung and was offered the opportunity to take chemotherapy. Dad had never before choked up in front of me, but that day he tearfully asked me if I could love a "bald old man."

His reaction to the possibility of chemotherapy scared me. Dad always had a plan in place, whether for family vacations or fishing trips with his friends, the best path to buying a new car or house, or the journey to retirement, paved with life insurance and CD savings. Then he followed the map he had so carefully created, and everything turned out fine. However, cancer blindsided him. A sudden onslaught of coughing brought him home early from a vacation in Branson, Missouri, with Mom, Aunt Bettye, and Uncle Hank. He traveled to Ohio in search of a more positive medical opinion. By the time he turned down palliative chemo (as I would later do after my own terminal diagnosis), he was almost too weak to fly home to Florida. With Bart as Dad's caregiver, they flew to Orlando, enjoying a rare upgrade to first class because Dad couldn't walk more than a few steps from a wheelchair. I drove Mom on a 15-hour trip from Northwest Ohio to her and Dad's house on Lake Griffin, where Dad's new boat was moored at the end of the dock. The journey home was Dad's last trip. He realized that, even with a wheelchair and assistance, he could never leave the house again, even to walk down the dock to his long-dreamed-of speedboat.

With these experiences flashing like huge "Don't let this happen to you!!!" neon warnings, I decided that I would go as far as fast as I could. In my head, Ian McKellen-as-Gandalf stridently commanded, "Fly, you fools!" (*The Lord of the Rings: The Fellowship of the Ring*), just as he had urged the Fellowship to flee an unstoppable fire monster, the Balrog. If Dad and Bart had fallen from battle with the Balrog of cancer, their unexpectedly swift decline spurred me to action. I fled, as Gandalf-in-my-head urged, but also physically flew—first to Iceland, later to Europe.

My plans during the first months after diagnosis were to live much as Queen Latifah's character, Georgia Bird, does in *Last Holiday* (2006) after she learns she has a terminal illness. She decides to spend all her money on a lavish vacation in a European hotel. Her millionaire lifestyle (for at least a few weeks) includes spa treatments, a new wardrobe, extreme sports, and gourmet delights. Her last holiday changes her from an introverted career worker to an extroverted explorer. Even when she receives word that she was misdiagnosed and is not about to die, she isn't bitter about splurging financially or spending time contemplating her mortality. Instead, she takes a chance on love and a new career—and gets the proverbial happy rom-com ending.

Although life for anyone is seldom a rom-com, I resist the mental temptation to fantasize about receiving a similar last-minute "Sorry, equipment malfunction—you'll outlive your savings" fax (or, more modernly, text) that allows me to happily push fears of dying out of the way for, say, another decade. However, living Bird's fantasy life of spending the money once so carefully saved for a far-off dreamy future is the part of the film that stands out in my mind years after seeing it in a cinema, and this plot conceit fueled my flights of fantasy and in reality.

My initial problem with taking several long trips was not my desire to leave or a lack of funds. Whenever I am asked about my finances, my glib reply has been "I'm spending Heather's inheritance." Balancing what I retain for medical expenses or leave in cash to my beneficiaries versus how much I spend on travel is an ongoing concern, especially as the economy fluctuates and my retirement stock accounts dwindle with every Dow plunge. What stopped me from making travel plans the day I received my terminal diagnosis, however, was not finances but time— I had just begun teaching courses scheduled for a 15-week semester. With my oncologist saying in January that I could have six months to live, I immediately latched onto that number, deleting anything past May (when, I calculated, I would still be mobile) from my mental calendar. Because classes were scheduled to end early in May, I wondered if I, like Dad and Bart, wouldn't be able to take one last vacation or a long-dreamed-of trip. Only the Wonder Women in my life spinning into action by taking over my work responsibilities allowed me to switch from teacher to tourist. Just as I had done for much of my life, I hit the road.

Even before Bart was born (in 1960), I was a road warrior. At two years old, I drove my tiny metal car up and down the gravel driveway of our brick ranch that Dad helped build on North Ruston Avenue in Evansville. At that time, the paved road that fronted our house ended at a barbed wire fence keeping the homeowners in the new subdivision from the grazing cows. My favorite part of the house surprisingly wasn't my pink bedroom but the carport beyond the back door. The reason was simple: I could make sweeping turns in my blue convertible or sometimes go round and round on the carport's concrete, especially on rainy days when the drive became muddy and puddled. Under supervision on warm afternoons, I even wheeled down the road to watch the cows.

Around that time, my parents started what would become a series of almost-annual spring treks to Florida. When Dad began selling insurance for Western-Southern Life, he worked hard to "make convention"— or be invited as one of the company's sales leaders to the annual business gathering, which, for decades, was held at the Fontainebleau Hotel in Miami Beach. Mom always said she felt better with a tan, and the convention usually was held in April—the perfect time to forget about winter snows in Indiana. My parents and I shared February birthdays—Dad's on the 11th, Mom's on the 22nd, mine on the 27th. Birthday celebrations helped make the grey skies of February bearable until the convention list was announced at the end of the month and, as a result of long hours far more than luck, my father's name was on it. From then until we packed our swimsuits, we all looked forward to April and Florida!

For me, that meant riding in the backseat of our '56 blue-and-white Chevy. I was too short to see anything but tall billboards out my window, so Mom focused my attention on workbooks that taught numbers and letters. As I rode, I "studied" so that, when I turned five, I would be ahead of the other kindergartners. I first learned to read by memorizing billboards and, upon arriving in Jacksonville for a visit with Aunt

Irene and Uncle Bart, astounded them when I pointed to a billboard advertising bread and correctly "read" the slogan.

On these earliest trips, I became a proficient junior traveler. My wooden potty chair fit on the floorboard in the backseat. In the late 1950s and early 1960s, rest parks along highways were practically non-existent, and off ramps did not lead to a plethora of fast-food restaurants. My parents didn't make frequent stops during the long drive. We ate a picnic-basketful of sandwiches during the long drive but drank very little juice or coffee. By three years old, I was an old hand at riding for hours in the car with books or "work" to entertain me and carefully timing my potty breaks.

When Bart was born, I gained a backseat travel companion. I sat on the right, behind Mom. Bart's seat was on the left, behind Dad, who always drove. *National Lampoon's Vacation* (1983) parodied our life as summer travelers, although Dad would have memorized Wally World's dates and hours of operation and never arrived when it was closed. By 1965, Dad earned two weeks of vacation time each summer, and, on the day school let out in June, the four of us climbed into the family car (which was—no joke—a woody station wagon) and headed west. As a child, Dad had few toys and especially prized his ViewMaster with a set of slides showing Garden of the Gods in Colorado. Thus, our '65 tour first covered Colorado before dipping into New Mexico to see the Painted Desert and Petrified Forest before heading northwest to Arizona's Grand Canyon and across more desert to Anaheim, California— and Disneyland! After tackling the theme park's Matterhorn, we drove to Yosemite National Park to view real mountains. In subsequent trips west we visited Yellowstone and Glacier National Parks. While everyone else in the country watched Neil Armstrong land on the moon, I was trying to figure out the pulley flush tank in our ancient cabin in Glacier. We had no television but didn't miss one because we were busy avoiding bears and hiking through fields of flowers by day and falling asleep early each night. Only when we were ready to leave the park and read a news-paper headline did we learn of (hu)mankind's giant leap.

Dad enjoyed showing us Canada, too. On other long vacations, our family flew in to fishing camps in Ontario or Quebec, catching and eat-ing what we caught until the plane arrived a week later to return us to "civilization." We toured Toronto, Ottawa, and Montreal on our drives either coming or going from fish camps. On a drive across much of Canada one summer, we visited Winnipeg on the way to Calgary and the Stampede, then headed to Banff (another of my favorite places) and Lake Louise, as well as took scenic drives through the Canadian Rockies.

Before I was graduated from high school, our family vacations had taken me to all states in the continental United States. Soon after Dad died, Mom looked to me as a travel companion on a tour of Alaska and northwestern Canada. When I conducted research about the television series *LOST* in 2005, I visited Oahu for the first time. Thus, I finally had visited every state in the United States—an achievement that would have made Dad proud. He taught me how to plan a trip and how and why to love traveling, and, as an adult, I became a true road (and plane) warrior by conducting research for books and presenting conference papers as a way to justify (or help pay for) my travels within and beyond the United States. Although I idolized the true traveler, Anthony Bourdain, for his adventures more than his cooking, I never achieved that level of connection with international cultures, and that is probably the one regret I take to my grave. However, I have logged a lot of miles in my lifetime.

Jen teases that I am her travel agent, but there is much truth in her jest. I like to control the process of making travel arrangements and enjoy comparing flights, layover times, and percentages of on-time flights. I look for the best amenities within our price range and bring along a list of restaurants, music venues, art galleries, and tours we might try. I study the history of an area (if I haven't visited before). During our years as travel buddies, Jen has been surprised but pleased by some of my detours. After we gave our conference presentations in Albuquerque, I rented a car, booked a hotel in Santa Fe, and drove the Turquoise Trail to get there. I introduced her to the mountains and deserts in a small section of New Mexico, explaining bits of tribal histories and stopping to take photos all along the way. The side trip made the conference even more educational and gave us more bonding time.

I also have learned from Jen. She operates in her own time zone, and I am the nag who keeps prodding her to get to the airport more than the required two hours ahead of flight time. Following a Honolulu conference on a trip in which I also introduced her to the beauty of North Shore, Waimea Valley, and the coastline near the Kualoa Ranch,

Jen decided there was no point sweating out the late-day flight at the airport or hanging around the hotel in our travel clothes. She booked a whale-watching tour for our final morning in Honolulu. I wasn't completely useless—I checked our bags at the hotel and later secured a room where travelers can change clothes and relax a couple of hours before heading to the airport. From this experience I began adding even more to my travel agenda, although I have to reassure myself that I will still make it to the airport in plenty of time for a flight.

In January 2018, when I heard that I might have as few as six months to live, and once my classes were covered, my skills as a "travel agent" became key to my success. Within two weeks of diagnosis, I scheduled flights to and from Reykjavik, Iceland; tours to the massive, mostly-frozen Gullfoss waterfall and the steamy sulfuric bubbles of the Geysir geyser field; a ticket to hear the Iceland Symphony Orchestra; and, following the advice of my ophthalmologist, who recommended a "Blue Lagoon sandwich," visiting the hot springs after the flight in and just before the flight out, booked a spa day. Another item on my to-do list concerned my wardrobe. Living in Florida means that my "winter wear" consists of a light jacket and a couple of long-sleeved shirts. Fortunately, Joy suggested places in central Florida where I could buy a ski-rated hooded coat, thermal base clothes, waterproof boots, and ski pants. When I finally crunched across frozen tundra or skated on icy patches near Gullfoss and Geysir, I looked like Ralphie's brother Randy in his snowsuit (*A Christmas Story*, 1983), but I was warm.

Iceland allowed me to appreciate that "otherness" can be empowering and healing. Seven hours after leaving Orlando, the plane landed early in the morning at Keflavik Airport. Because of the limited hours of sunlight in Iceland in early March, the sun gradually bathed the black-and-white landscape in pale pink light during the hour-long bus ride into Reykjavik. Feeling more like a Starfleet visitor to a distant planet than a tourist in Iceland, I stared at the long stretches of black volcanic rock leading toward snow-crested mountains. On subsequent day tours from Reykjavik, I peered out bus windows at rural farms identified by white clouds pointing to their geothermal heat source and looked for the short, sturdy Iceland horses in pastures. The plains between mountains suddenly revealed a slash where the mighty series of Gullfoss cascades, shrouded in sheets of ice, roared through rock.

At Geysir I alternated holding a gloved hand over my frosty nose (the only uncovered part of my face) and poising my trigger finger on my camera while I awaited a geyser's performance. Although it occurs approximately every 10 minutes, those minutes stretched infinitely when my nose or finger risked frostbite. When the geyser shot a stream of water about 20 feet high, I oohed and aahed as I snapped photos. The sulfuric spray immediately blew across half of the circle of tourists standing remarkably close. Fortunately, I had heeded my guide's suggestion to stand on the opposite side, with the wind to my back.

Icelanders seem to believe that tourists are smart enough to figure out these things. They also seem to expect visitors will not walk to the icy edge of a chasm, turn around, and lean back to take a selfie or to fall into scalding water in a geyser field. Few physical barriers separate humans and nature, which surprised and pleased me, even as I recognized that litigious-minded Americans would take advantage of this common sense approach to safety.

Whether in my Reykjavik hotel or at the Blue Lagoon, I took advantage of the tamer hot pools. At the Hilton, an English-speaking attendant explained that, if I entered the first pool, a masseuse would join me to massage my neck and shoulders. A second pool invited me to cool off before I walked outside to a cedar sauna or an open-air hot pool, its clouds of steam obscuring the cold morning sky. Because women and men were segregated at the spa, nudity was encouraged. Because I was the only non–Icelandic speaker on the day I visited, I resorted to mime and a lot of smiling and nodding when women tried to engage me in conversation. Both experiences are outside my comfort zone but great fodder for jokes—I hope other bathers laughed with me, not at me, but I will never know.

At the Blue Lagoon, I heard many languages spoken, but English-speaking attendants guided me through the locker and shower rooms to the connected series of outdoor pools. I swam out of the shower area directly into the lagoon. Because of a double-digit temperature difference between the water and air, steamy clouds obscured other bathers until we were inches apart. Even the sun was just a bright smudge overhead, mostly hidden by shifting wisps or waves of clouds. Adding to the surreality of this setting was a very popular swim-up bar, where I used my credit wristband to buy cool, fruity drinks that I sipped while stretching out on rocky ledges mostly submerged in hot water.

Considering my bathing attire, I turned away the swimming photographer who offered to capture the spa day for posterity. The Blue Lagoon's milky blue pools have a high silica content, and the lava rocks surrounding the lagoon are covered with layers of white silica. To avoid silica getting into my hair and making it stiff and probably a new color, I wore a tight white cap pulled over my ears and ear plugs. My glasses, coated with a solution provided in the shower area that kept the lenses clear, were perched outside my rubber-covered ears. Everything but my silica-proofed head lurked below the water line most of the time, adding to my sense of being an alien in a completely new environment. Bathers floating by probably agreed that I seemed alien, someone foreign in every sense of the word.

Even taking a city tour of Reykjavik proved to be strangely challenging and unexpectedly entertaining. When the tour van stopped for a brief visit to Hallgrímskirkja, a Lutheran church with an imposingly towered façade that can be seen from just about everywhere in town, I decided to instead get a latte at Loki's Café across the street. Only the day before, I'd spent more than an hour climbing the tower and photographing the view from each open window at the top. As is my custom when I visit a religious site, I meditated. The high-arched nave afforded me a quiet, safe space to stop and inwardly listen before I resumed my tour. Warming up with a latte seemed a much better option on the second day of touring Reykjavik. However, I wanted to make sure the driver knew where I was headed and that I had enough time to visit Loki's before the van would depart. "Thor," I asked (seriously, that was his name), "do I have time to go to Loki's?" As a Marvel fan fond of film-version Thor (Chris Hemsworth) and Loki (Tom Hiddleston), I had to ask that question. Thor, who probably hears a lot of similar questions from fan-tourists, warned me to be back in 10 minutes. I happily trotted across the street to the little café named for the shapeshifting Norse god.

As soon as I ordered the latte in English but prepared to point to the menu in lieu of a translator, the barista asked where in the States was home. My hands as much as my language and accent gave me away. Although I lotioned faithfully, I frequently removed my gloves while taking a photo, and even brief exposure to the cold air dried and cracked my hands, which were unused to such weather. While the milk was being steamed, the barista shared a glop of lotion that she promised would protect my hands all day; she used it to keep hers soft and moisturized. Thanking her, I spread the lotion across both palms and made sure to cover my hands thoroughly, not realizing that the thick, creamy lotion was mostly lanolin—slippery, absorbent, almost-pure lanolin— the stuff that protects Iceland's sheep from rain or snow. I picked up the recyclable cup of frothy latte with both hands to warm them, sipped appreciably, thanked the barista again, and walked to the door with three minutes to spare before Thor drove off. True to Loki's nature as a trickster, the brass door knob could not be turned. First one hand, then the other, without glove or with, slipped as I tried to open the door. Finally, a kind (and probably inwardly laughing) Icelander standing outside the café noticed my plight and opened the door for me. Pretending cold and not embarrassment colored my cheeks red, I hastily thanked him and ran for the van. I was the last one on, but Thor was kind enough not to smirk as, latte firmly braced with two hands, I took my seat.

Days like these remind me how "American" and "other" I am, even in a country used to international tourists. However, on this trip, I felt out of my element because I experienced a new geography and culture, not because I have cancer. People made assumptions about me based on my appearance—but these preconceptions were related to cultural differences, not medical ones. Some guides addressed me in German or Swedish, thinking I "look" European. In a hot pool or at the symphony, locals spoke to me in Icelandic, looking surprised when I pantomimed my guess at answering or sadly admitted that I only speak English. Iceland reaffirmed my need to leave my comfort zone in a positive way. Whereas Iceland proved to be enlightening, exciting, and empowering because it is different from anyplace else I have traveled, a trip to Scandinavia offered more challenges, most often because of the ways that other tourists or the cruise ship's well-meaning crew perceived me.

It has been said that travel "broadens the mind," but it also makes one aware of one's limitations and preconceptions. In my case, solo travel also has forced me to face the realities of how others perceive me and how their expectations for my appearance, behavior, and lifestyle reflect the ways many people have been conditioned to think of (1) single women, (2) senior women, and (3) the terminally ill. However, my Scandinavian vacation helped me understand my actual versus expected place in the world. In short, I became more aware of others' expectations or preconceptions but didn't let them stop me. My only concern is that this independent attitude may work against me someday when my deteriorating physical condition means I really should have assistance. As a "dead" woman, I must be aware of how my body is faring each day and realistically plan my activities—with or without assistance—so as not to move from "dead" to dead even faster.

A few entries from my travel diary illustrate my surprise at seeing myself through others' eyes. On July 4, the ship docked in Hamburg, Germany, on a morning when fog delayed the first tour groups disembarking the ship. As a result, I even more eagerly than usual hopped onto the tour bus for an overview of the city before some free time in the city center. I summarized the excursion this way.

On the tour I saw the highlights of the warehouse district, the red light district (where the Beatles got their start in clubs), and numerous churches, including Michel—although I had a tough time taking the photo I wanted of St. Michael's statue. [I feel especially fond of him because I was taught in Reiki classes (Reiki is an energy-channeling healing technique) to ask for his protection and grounding blue light and because, if I'd been male, I would have been named Michael.] I envied the Germans strolling around Alster Lakes on this blue-skied summer day. Bustling City Hall fascinated me because of its ornate architecture; almost every inch serves an artistic purpose. Among the tourists jockeying for the best spot for a photo of the immense building are street performers. My eyes kept returning to the mime clowns, whose antics intrigued me as well as seemed a wee bit creepy.

When we were given two hours of freedom on the "on your own" part of the tour before the tour buses returned to the ship, I prepared to scamper off to Alster Lakes. My plan was to walk at least partway around them before time ran out and I had to return to the bus. However, as I moved away from the group, a tour guide from the cruise line stopped me. "Where is your partner?" she worriedly asked. I thought she had mistaken me for someone else, although, with my purple-and-red hair, that was difficult to do. "I'm on my own," I replied and turned to leave, thinking the conversation was over. "Where are you going?" the guide persisted. I explained the Alster Lakes plan, much to her concern. "I'm not sure that's a good idea," she began, and I asked whether the area, even on this sunny morning, was crime ridden. "No, that's not it," she shook her head. "What if you fall or get lost? I don't mean you're old, but what if you can't get back to the ship? I don't like to see a woman your age go off on her own." Trying to hide my irritation, because Mom taught me that if I can't say anything nice, not to say anything at all, I assured the guide that I would only walk as far as I could still see the bridge as my landmark to the central city and would be careful. Still, with her eyes on me even after I crossed the street and admired the view, I aborted my plan to walk very far. I took a brief stroll partway around a lake before returning to City Hall. As I meandered through its archway into a back courtyard, I photographed the many stained glass zodiac signs and plaster gods and an ornate fountain. Next, I ambled a few blocks to St. Nicolai and photographed the church's lion door knockers—the oldest remaining art in the city [which was heavily bombed during World War II]. I shopped in a bookstore and, afterward, bought a slab of kuchen in a bakery. Even in a small way, I wanted to sample Hamburg away from the ship or bus. Although I enjoyed my free time, I didn't feel as free as usual—and I wondered if the tour guide knew more than she was telling or if I overestimate my ability to take care of myself.

Although I did ride the bus back to the ship, I quickly ditched my "old lady" cardi and decided to leave the ship to walk through the warehouse district and down to the harbor. I ultimately chickened out from walking in the tunnel under the Elbe in favor of walking beside the river. I decided to buy a Hamburg Hard Rock t-shirt, both as an homage to the Beatles' early career in the city and to my wardrobe 30 years ago that largely consisted of Hard Rock t-shirts from a variety of cities. The new shirt is red like my hair and fiery like my stubborn independence. Up on the roof bar, I relished the shade and breeze on this sultry day and quietly watched the river. Hard Rock was packed with German tourists, and my point-and-smile method of ordering rum and Cokes and cheese fries made everyone aware that I did not speak the language. Although that earned me a few side-eyes from people seated around me, I didn't keep their attention long. All of a sudden the rooftop patrons pointed and excitedly shouted as they rushed to get a better view of the Elbe. The *Louisville*, an old-fashioned paddle-wheeler, tooted its steam whistle and began chugging down the river. I'm used to seeing paddleboats, from my trips to New Orleans and hometown on the Ohio, but this type of boat obviously is a novelty in Hamburg. For once, something familiar to me, a foreigner, was "touristy" to the locals.

Although the rum and cheese fries made me walk faster on my way back to the ship and my independent walks through tourist-heavy areas of central Hamburg during daylight hardly seemed risky, I felt the ridiculous need to "prove" that I am still a careful, observant, and time-conscious single tourist who doesn't need (and often doesn't want) a tour partner.

Similarly, I embraced my free time in Oslo. After a tour of the Munch Museum and a special viewing of "The Scream" in the National Museum, I returned to the central city to experience the Pride parade. According to my travel diary, I "sang and danced with locals on the sidelines as the floats slowly passed and enjoyed being part of the crowd." I savored rainbow-colored ice cream and, full and warm, sat in a park. Like so many others lounging along the waterfront, I lifted my face to the sun and felt the rays soak into my pores. (Melanoma from overexposure to sun is not a big concern for me these days.) As I noted in the diary, this was probably the only time during the entire vacation where no one in the world knew exactly where I was at that moment, and I was OK with that.

Although I logically understood that summer days so far north in the Northern Hemisphere last very long, I still marveled at sunrise on the sea's horizon around 4:30 at the northernmost point of our voyage. Often I ordered coffee by 5:00 so that I could sit on the balcony and think or write for a few hours before the day's tours began. An entry written early on July 5, as I enjoyed the first sun rays and first coffee from my balcony, illustrates my continuing reflection of others' expectations of women like me.

> So many people have commented on my traveling alone. On the Danish castle tour, my lunch companions [a group of women about my age] called me "brave" and "inspiring" to take a cruise on my own. I don't understand that. I realize many people have family or work responsibilities that limit their time to travel. Lots of people don't have the money to do so. (I feel like a poor tourist compared to those who tell me they take at least six cruises a year, they've been on this ship three times so far, or they aren't bothering to get off the ship this time because they've been to this destination so many times.) My enthusiasm for briefly visiting new cities, especially the small ones, or walking through the countryside or along a beach is only enhanced by the simplicity of a life on board. Cruises are easy—I'm herded from place to place off the ship. My meals and wine are provided. I'm told the temperature and what to take or wear ashore. I don't see anything "brave" or "inspiring" about it. It's just a lot of fun! [If my health issues had created an obvious public problem for me or others, perhaps I might have understood why they applauded my single travel. They were astonished that a woman of my age wanted and could travel solo.]
>
> I was also surprised by the kindly crew member who assisted tour guides on the day trip to Skagen, Denmark. On our way back to the ship, the only vacant seat on the bus was next to me. "Is anyone going to sit next to you?" the young man asked. I smiled. "Only you." He returned the smile and sat down. "So your husband stayed on the ship?" he casually inquired (and I knew he was making conversation and not chatting me up). "I'm single," I said. "But you were married, right? Just no husband right now?" "No," I assured him, "no husband past or present. I like traveling alone." He frowned. "Aren't you sad to see all the other couples? Don't you miss having a family?" Once again, I gently reassured him that I was not sad or lonely. In fact, I like being able to do what I want, when I want. "I'm sorry if I've overstepped," he apologized, "but I just think it's so sad that you're alone." Because I have never let my single status keep me from traveling, I forget that most of the world wants to see people paired up, and the heteronormative world expects a woman to have a husband. If I were widowed or divorced (from anyone,

irrespective of gender), I could be more understandable because, at least, I once was part of a duo, a couple, a partnership. Being never married in my 60s and, apparently to this young man, desirable enough that I could be expected to have been married—or at least be having a tryst on board—presented an unfathomable situation.

Although another scenario didn't even warrant a diary entry, I recall the miscommunication between a restaurant host and me early in the voyage. I reserved a table for one at the ship's most exclusive restaurant. When I arrived a few minutes before the reservation time, the host checked my name in her book and asked me to be seated. I thought nothing of this until several couples or small groups were taken to their table before me, and my reservation time passed. I walked to the host stand to ask, "Will I be seated soon?" The host looked surprised. "Just as soon as your companion arrives," she explained. Shaking my head, I said I was dining alone and had made the reservation for one. She explained that she thought I had just clicked the wrong number online, because no one dines alone. "I do," I emphasized, whereby she apologized and led me to a window table set for two. Before my starter arrived, I had to confirm with two servers that I was enjoying a meal by myself, the extra place setting could be removed, and no one else would arrive later. After that rigmarole, however, the service was impeccable, and the French cuisine superb. I have seldom enjoyed a solo dining experience more.

Lest I give the impression that the Scandinavian cruise vacation only tested my resolve as a solo traveler, even without being aware that this may be one of, if not my last overseas trips or agonizing over what my digestive system might be doing at any given moment, here are two representative diary entries from an amazing 10 days at sea or on shore. Especially in Skagen, Denmark, I was just another tourist, like everyone else on the tour.

> I am so glad I chose the seascapes excursion [in Skagen]! We were bused past two old lighthouses—a white wooden replica of the 1600s model and the actual grey brick lighthouse in a style like Ponce Inlet's [a lighthouse a few miles from my Florida home]. A much older (1400s) first lighthouse could be seen on a hill far from today's beach. This early model consists of a basket-and-pulley mechanism; a bucket of fire was hoisted maybe 30 feet in the air as a warning to sailors. With the treacherous waters at the spit of land where the North and Baltic Seas meet, it's no wonder that the map of shipwrecks is called a "caviar map," full of dark dots close together.

I rode a "sandworm"—a tractor-pulled wagon that shouldn't get stuck in the dunes' and beaches' loose sand. The North Sea side is losing several feet in height, which the Baltic Sea side is gaining every year. Just as the many lighthouses' locations chart the coastline's changes, so do daily photographs in a local museum show how much the wind and sea alter the coastline all the time.

Despite all the sand, the beach is surprisingly rocky. Lots of colorful pebbles wash up all the time. I need to identify the sparkly grey, red, brown, and white stones I collected to give to the kids back home. Of course, I pulled off my trainers so I could wade in the cold water. I've now stuck my toes in two seas at once!

The next stop was at a nature center explaining the area's geology and geography. Before we arrived at the center, which stands alone in an area of sand and scrub brush, the guide warned us to watch out for "wipers" when we walked up the path. It was a hot afternoon, so I immediately envisioned people jumping at us to wipe our sweaty brows as soon as we stepped off the bus—kind of like Toronto's squeegee people who come out of nowhere to wash your car's windscreen while you're stopped at a light. It took a few minutes to realize the guide was saying *vipers*—the poisonous adders who come out on warm days to sun. From then on, I stomped up and down the paths so that the snakes would easily feel the vibrations and stay away.

On the last day of the cruise, we docked in Amsterdam, a city I quickly adored during my first three-day visit a few years earlier, when I spent much of my time at the Rijksmuseum and the Van Gogh Museum. That summer I researched and wrote a book about the way Van Gogh has been portrayed in popular culture, kind of a myth versus fact book. One of my favorite places in the world is the Van Gogh Museum, and, although I knew I would only have a brief visit this time, I longed to see "Vincent" again. Of that visit I wrote,

The museum has expanded since I last was here, but much of the original exhibition space is still familiar. I rushed to see a few of my favorite paintings, such as "Almond Blossom," "Tree Roots," and "Wheatfield with Crows." Although I know that "Tree Roots," rather than "Wheatfield with Crows," is most likely Van Gogh's final painting, I nonetheless teared up in front of "Wheatfield," not out of sorrow for the dark skies and ominous crows but in relief and joy that I was there—right in front of the art that Van Gogh painted, his brushstrokes still evident after all these years. I was standing in Amsterdam, so far from my start in Indiana, admiring this master's art—and I had been fortunate enough to see it not once in my lifetime, but twice. On an art high after an hour in the museum—and thankful that I had bought my ticket weeks earlier online so that I could be allowed to see Van Gogh's paintings and sketches on a "sold out" day—I walked down the center of the Museumplein to absorb the energy of the museum crowds, people walking in the

park on a Saturday, and sunbathers stretched out on the grass. This is timeless. This is life, and I soak it in.

Although these entries may seem undesirably passive to many read-
ers, I admit that I have never been interested in extreme sports. My tour
"activities" often include walking around museums or art galleries,
strolling rather than climbing (even though 20 years ago I nervously
but successfully climbed narrow steps to the tops of Mayan temples),
or sitting in a theatre. Nonetheless, they represent who I am. Cancer
may have encouraged an even more sedentary lifestyle, especially at certain points of my treatment or after surgeries. However, I have never
been athletic and often seek out the historic or the beautiful instead of
the heart pounding or adrenalin fueled.

Because I visited countries I had not previously visited or had seen
only briefly—Denmark, Sweden, Norway, Germany, and the Netherlands—this trip became far more than a checked item on my bucket list.
It offered natural beauty, the great art of Edvard Munch and Vincent
van Gogh, new foods to taste, and new cities to explore. However, it
also afforded me the time to analyze my identity, past and present, in
comparison with others' preconceptions. This trip is part of a much
longer life voyage and prompted a reconnection with the parts of me
that I like best—my enthusiasm for more experience, my love of the
arts, and my openness to being spiritually healed by nature.

In the months since I returned from my momentous international
travels, I returned to work and became more geographically limited to
weekend travels or University-sanctioned conference or research trips.
If I have learned anything in life, it is to listen to my instincts and, if I
feel something is important to do—whether it makes sense to anyone
else—I do it. I try not to put off until tomorrow what I can do today—
an adage that applies to play as much as work. Just getting out of the
house for a few hours on a weekend can be restorative, especially when
I wander along Ormond or Daytona Beach, see explosions of color from
the azaleas in nearby Ravine Gardens State Park, dance to Albannach's
pounding drums at a Celtic festival, or watch the bees at an apiary.

At times, I have ventured out of state for small conferences or
research. In September I participated in a writers' conference in Albuquerque, where I met author Anne Hillerman. Her father, Tony, wrote
a series of Navajo detective novels that Anne has continued, a series

that I have reread a few times. In November I studied a Georgia O'Keeffe exhibition in Raleigh, North Carolina. During the academic year I participated more actively in popular culture conferences in New Orleans and Chicago. Life is not only what but where I make it, which is why I embrace the much-used metaphor of life being a journey (or a story of a journey). My current cancer journey is only one leg of a much more important and longer life journey featuring thousands of interesting stops or side trips. When I no longer can physically travel, I will mentally return to the places I have explored or share one of my travel diaries so my friends can tell more tales about me.

CHAPTER 6

Taking Care of Business

Not all of my post-prognosis planning involved lengthy vacations to places I always wanted to see. I also had to take care of business at home as part of my pre-death master plan. The business of dying—or planning for death—takes time and money. Whole industries surround the dying, starting with medical interventions and maintenance and ending with legal disbursement of everything from the corpse to the deceased's possessions and leftover debts. I may joke that I can't take it with me, but that's the truth, so the choice for the soon-to-be-dead is what to do between knowing that death is imminent and deciding what to do with that knowledge.

A colleague in my department seemed awestruck when I explained that I already had a will and beneficiaries designated for my bank accounts and insurance policies but now urgently wanted to take care of more details—such as deciding what will happen to my mementos with only sentimental value or decluttering my home quickly. He said that his father wanted to leave all those decisions to his children; he preferred to spend his time enjoying his home and not worrying about what would happen after his death. After all, he wouldn't care after death. That was a valid choice for him, but it differs from mine. The longer I live, the more I vacillate between agonizing over every last detail and realizing that my colleague's father is correct—I won't care what happens to my body or my things once I am gone. However, until the moment I die, I will want to make my passing as easy as possible on my family and friends.

Perhaps my urgency to take care of all the business of dying is the result of my parents' work ethic and meticulous planning. They carefully kept folders marked by type of payment or receipt in the lower right desk drawer. They set up wills and powers of attorney well in advance of final illnesses. Dad made sure all his business accounts were ready to be smoothly transferred to Mom, and Mom equally divided her estate between Bart and me.

Although I am far less precise (I organize by stack on my desk or periodically add paperwork to an "everything" folder of legal documents), at least I have pulled together the deed to my burial plot in Indiana, the account numbers for insurance policies and bank accounts, my latest tax returns, and notes about payments to everyone from my homeowners' association or life insurance company down to the quarterly gutter cleaners or the florists who beautify my parents' graves. However, when I received my prognosis, I wanted to make even more precise decisions not only about spreading my ashes on land and sea but also spreading my influence as far as possible. For me, the business of dying is separate from the business of death, yet both are important and require far more finesse than I ever expected.

The business of dying involves my wishes about how I wish to be treated medically—or not—and where and how I prefer to die. Fortunately, my close friends Jen and Joy are on literally the same page, page 8 of the will that lists them as administrators of my wishes and guardians if or when I become incapacitated. About a year before my cancer diagnosis, I was prompted by Bart's terminal illness to make a new will; an old one created by a "will shop" as soon as I relocated to Florida just wasn't adequate for my current situation. As my advising attorney, Joy knows how to prepare a will, but she, Jen, and I needed to sit down and go over details so that she could prepare the documents for signing. The afternoon meeting around Joy's kitchen table turned raucous as we joked about my choices and comments—I doubt if anyone has had so much fun in preparing a will. A week or so later, Joy, Jen, and I attended a National Theatre Live screening—something we and Joy's and Jen's mother Lynn have always enjoyed sharing. Watching a filmed play at the little Enzian theatre in Maitland while we eat and drink—then discussing the play and our lives during the interval or afterward—is our special time together. At this Enzian get-together, Joy brought the final copies of the will to be signed, and, before the lights dimmed, we signed multiple pages and made my future secure. Creating a will was just something I needed to do, but the process was not fraught with anxiety.

On the contrary, it was a lot of fun and provided us with another excuse to socialize.

After my short-term prognosis, I had to think even more seriously about what would happen longer term: after my death. During the creation of the earlier will, I had a vision of some far-off day when, in my 90s, I might fall and hit my head, requiring Jen to sign hospital documents so I could be treated. When I died as the oldest (formerly) living professor in Florida, Joy might have to take my death certificate to the bank to get into my safe deposit box. Whereas, just a few years ago, agreeing to be my power of attorney or executor of my will seemed to be no big deal, now those tasks assume immense importance. They likely will involve decisions about whether I can remain at home until death or need to receive constant supervision. My friends will decide how best to use funds in my bank accounts to pay for my care or serve as a trustee to disburse funds to creditors and inheritors. Now the stakes are much higher, and the necessary decisions will take place much sooner. Nevertheless, Jen and Joy still agreed to sign on for the difficult times ahead.

Len Wein, who co-created Marvel's Wolverine among his many gifts to comics, is credited with a lovely and accurate quotation about friendship: "A true friend is someone who is there for you when he'd rather be anywhere else." I prefer to make this statement plural and gender neutral, but it acknowledges what I often forget about my death, lingering or not— Jen and Joy (and, I hope only half in jest, at least a dozen but preferably thousands) will be saddened by my loss. Although their future grief is difficult for me to accept and causes me pain, no matter how glib I seem on the surface, I do want to be remembered, especially fondly.

Even when I received bad news about a rectal tumor discovered during a colonoscopy back in April 2016, I tried to make Jen less sad, but I still felt terrible about causing her tears. After we left the doctor's office, we ended up sharing sandwiches on my couch while I joked about planning my "make a wish" moments or benefitting from the perks of cancer (e.g., Could I be wheeled to the front of the lines at Universal before as well as during chemo? Could my extended family spend time with me at the beach right before my surgery, so I could go swimming with them before having an ileostomy? Could someone alert Benedict Cumberbatch's agents that I would appreciate a get well message from him?). Then Jen and I more stoically discussed the timeline for my treatments, rides to treatments, and temporary disability status instead of teaching during the fall semester. I seldom cry, but it's important to acknowledge others' tears before I plow ahead with how we are going to deal with my illness—and, throughout every moment, I try to express my gratitude that I don't have to figure out everything or go through cancer alone.

Similarly, soon after my terminal diagnosis, my extended family— Joy, Nico, Jen, Chris, Layla, Thomas, and Lynn—took me on a weekend trip to the Gulf coast. We stayed in Tampa to enjoy the hotel's amenities before making the short drive to Honeymoon Island State Park and taking a ferry to one of our favorite beaches at Caladesi Island. As Lynn and I lounged at the outside bar before dinner, I commented that I had thoroughly enjoyed playing with the kids in the pool and soaking until I pruned in the hot tub—and all that after strolling along the nearby boardwalk around and over a lake to watch the egrets and herons. It was a great day, and I mused that I couldn't believe my life was ending so soon and I wouldn't have many more of these days. (I also have a talent for beheading joyful, relaxed moments with my self-reflection.) Lynn noted that I seemed to be doing well, and I agreed, adding that the adults who knew seemed to be handling everything OK, too. Lynn shook her head. "Jenny is not taking this *at all* well," she told me. I was surprised, because Jen is most often stoic, pragmatic, and supportive when we are together. The few tears shed in my presence had fallen after the initial diagnosis and terminal follow-up. Although I highly recommend relying on the people one knows will be faithful to one's dying wishes and plans, I need to remind myself (and perhaps others) that agreeing to serve as a power of attorney, executor to a will, or trustee can be an emotionally rending task that becomes even more emotional when it comes time to fulfill those roles. I need to accept and plan for others' emotions as well as my own.

I also wanted to re-hear a quotation from *Third Star* (2010), a low-budget indie film that has helped me deal with the process of dying and death, first my relatives' and now mine. As a fan of Benedict Cumberbatch in the days after his initial *Sherlock* fame but before his Academy Award nomination or Marvel superhero role, I first saw this little Wales-set film in 2011 in London. In the following months, I helped bring it to my local Cinematique art cinema as part of the From Britain with Love series, and reviewed it and interviewed the director for *PopMatters*. A few years later, I returned to *Third Star* when Bart told me he had 18 months to live and when I was told I had six to possibly 12 months to live. The plot is simple—four friends take a final buddy road trip to Barafundle Bay, which is lead character James' favorite spot. Cumberbatch (James), as the young man dying from cancer, tells his estranged best friend, "I feared that nothing would go on without me. It's a relief to know that it will." I didn't understand that dialogue until I found out I was terminally ill. Until that point, I had first identified with Miles (JJ Feild), a workaholic whose father died of cancer and who can't bear seeing up close how his friend is dying. I regretted that I couldn't be Davy (Tom Burke), the caregiver who intimately knows all of James' medical and emotional vulnerabilities. After my terminal diagnosis, I began to identify with sometimes-preachy James, who tries to find meaning in each conversation with his friends and, against medical advice, goes adventuring one more time, even though he is often a burden to his friends. The world will go on without me—but my trust will still have to pay taxes, my condo will need to be sold, and the insurance and utilities paid until then. After I am gone, the business of living goes on for my "stuff" and the people entrusted to taking care of it. My friends and family will make new friends and face changes in their lives about which I will know nothing, and the world will continue changing. I only hope that I will have lived as fully as possible and done as good a job as possible to keep what remains of my little world revolving once I can no longer take care of things myself.

   Third Star also summarizes my expectations both of what it means to watch a loved one die *and* to be the dying loved one. The circumstances regarding my, Bart's, or Dad's terminal illness differ in the details, but we each have been a Davy, Miles, or James. Because I can better understand each character's response to death-inducing cancer, I try to be more aware of and sensitive to my friends' and family's emotions, even when they are hidden from my sight. They are now enacting Davy's or Miles' role.

   Not only choosing the people who may be in charge of me before I die but definitely will need to take charge of all I leave behind upon my death is only part of the weighty business required before I can rest in peace. The business of death involves not only me but all the stuff I have accumulated across six decades (even longer, if I count what I inherited from my parents and maternal grandmother). In addition to preparing a new will and a trust, I also must decide who gets what and distribute gifts, plan a memorial service and an obituary, figure out how to get rid of the body, and perhaps leave a legacy.

In March 2018, Joy and Carlos suggested that I talk with an attorney who specializes in wills and trusts. They made the connection for me and were great listeners when I developed a list of questions for the first meeting. On a beautiful April day, I drove the hour and a half to a cozy little office in Melbourne, just off the Intercoastal Waterway. Carlos and Joy made a fine recommendation—the attorney answered all my questions, drew up the papers to establish a trust with myself as the current trustee and two successors, created a new will and power of attorney forms, filed the paperwork to place my home under the trust, and, best of all, provided me with a folder of forms and instructions to ensure the appropriate financial accounts and documents came under the auspices of the trust. I also signed a living will that stipulates that no extraordinary measures will be taken to keep me alive. When my body is ready to go, my mind agrees it should be allowed, as comfortably as possible, to die. Instead of feeling sad for the need to file these papers or overwhelmed by my to-do list to finish creating the trust, I took a deep breath and relaxed for the first time in months. As *Third Star's* James said, life will go on without me, but I can help make sure the transition is easy, and, perhaps in a monetary way, I can help others benefit financially from my death. On the way home from Melbourne, I stopped for lunch at an outdoor seafood restaurant on the banks of the Intercoastal. Even the skies threatening rain couldn't dampen my mood; I was part of this natural cycle of sun and showers, and I could metaphorically embrace both.

Of course, nothing legal is ever easy; some institution or form is bound to cause concern, if not a downright difficult problem. I could complain about specific employees at a county department or a financial institution not caring about what, to me, is a matter of life and death. Business is not often speedy or as compassionate as I would like, but I also have to remember that the majority of people are sensitive and helpful. No one is ever going to be as emphatic as I about my need to have paperwork completed and filed appropriately, and few people may understand my heightened anxiety over everything being done correctly so there are no legal or procedural glitches after my death.

My experience with one local branch bank is a case in both the frustration and the relief in establishing a trust. When I initially tried to place my accounts within the trust, the branch bank employee setting up the trust demanded that I turn over the original documents to her— or else the bank could not even consider my request to change my accounts from my name to the trust's. After I explained that the original documents were kept at my attorney's office in Melbourne, she said I would have to get them and bring them in. (I later learned from a branch manager in Melbourne, my attorney, and another employee at my branch that this demand was incorrect.) When I got on the phone with my attorney as my frustration increased exponentially each minute, the bank employee would not talk with my attorney, stating that would be against bank policy. However, she could overhear my conversation with my attorney and shouted questions during the phone call. She also protested that she wasn't being difficult but only following bank policy. Finally, my attorney supported me when I said I could just take my money elsewhere or, at least, go to another branch. Finally, the bank employee accepted an emailed copy of the trust document, printed it, and said she would hand it to the appropriate legal representation for the bank. A few days later, I received a call to come to the branch and sign the papers. I thought everything was finally set up, and my successor trustee(s) and beneficiaries would have no trouble getting the money I set aside through the trust.

Thus, I was, in quick succession, surprised, dismayed, and angry when I found out six months later that some of my accounts that were supposedly included within the trust had not been. The paperwork to establish the trust had not been completed or filed by the bank employee who initiated the process in April. At that point, I testily mentioned to the woman currently helping me that this failure left the bank open to a lawsuit if one of my beneficiaries decided to challenge the way my money was supposed to be divided according to the trust's documentation. I apologized that this woman was hearing my ire when she had not created the problem. Nevertheless, I think I was justified in expecting that all employees should be able to do their job correctly. What would have happened if I had not lived longer than my prognosis of six months? What problems would the successor trustee(s) have had in following my wishes? Would my niece or friends have sought legal action against the bank? Although the bank representative who finally sorted out the mess (and confided that, as a result, she had found other accounts that hadn't been completed correctly) was kind and helpful, I still had to make two trips to the bank and be loudly indignant about my situation before the paperwork was filed correctly.

At least to me, the bank's expectation for me as a dying customer was for me to be grateful that my problem could be found and solved, but my demeanor should be rather passive if I wanted to succeed. Seldom do I express frustration vocally or show irritation with narrowed eyes or frown, but dealing with bureaucracy when I don't know if I will live long enough to spot a problem, much less correct it, even though I have done everything according to my attorney's instructions, is beyond mere frustration. It is demeaning and frightening.

On the day that I sat for two hours at the bank while the problems were unraveled, my increased anxiety and my body's general unpredictability led to my urgent need to use the restroom. On a previous branch visit to cash a check inside the bank, I had suffered a similar attack and, upon explaining my need to use the restroom, been told that it was only for employees. I had an accident in the lobby and had to drive home before I could clean up in a bathroom. Therefore, I panicked when I realized something similar could happen while the trust was being discussed, but this time I couldn't immediately drive home. Fortunately, the bank representative working with me was good with handling all sorts of trust issues. When I asked to use the restroom, she hastily unlocked the door to the hallway and the restroom, as well as told the nearest teller not to lock the door again until I left the bank. Saying I was relieved—in every sense of the word—throughout the rest of my long afternoon at the bank is the proverbial vast understatement. Still, in retrospect, I wonder whether I would have been given bathroom privileges if I had not already learned of the bank's error and hinted at the possibility of a future lawsuit.

That this was not the only obstruction to completing the to-do list created for me by my attorney is probably typical of any city's or state's bureaucracy, but that realization doesn't make any easier the long waits in offices, explanations of "we don't want to do it that way," or months of anxiety to find out if, indeed, the proper paperwork has been filed. However, if that is part of the business of dying, I can deal with it and the resulting anxiety, although it would be nice if some agencies' employees could empathize a little more. Perhaps the best advice I can give as a "dead" woman is to get a recommendation for and then "interview" an attorney specifically aware of state laws regarding trusts, estates, and wills. Then, after asking all questions and feeling confident that the attorney and documents are following one's directives and preferences, follow the attorney's advice. The objective is gaining peace of mind in order to rest (or work or play) in peace. The mandatory legal requirements for setting up a trust and putting everything important within it was far from my favorite task, but the relief at finally completing those chores was well worth the hours spent in waiting rooms. Being able to plan ahead as much as possible financially and medically for end-of-life care and the afterdeath is not always pleasant to contemplate, but someone has to deal with this reality. It might as well be me.

Although thinking about my life's finale while I am still able to work or travel is often difficult, I conversely enjoy planning the afterdeath celebration. By then, I will be out of pain, and the party can begin. A big focus of death, as traditionally commemorated by my relatives, is the funeral. I am not concerned about having one, but I want at least some type of acknowledgment of the death of my body and transition into something else, whether the pragmatism of ashes or a spiritual ascension into another dimension.

As a 2018 article in *The Economist* noted, "few choose how they die, but they can choose what happens next. Most leave this to loved ones who, in their distress, usually outsource the decision to an undertaker." Considering that the average funeral in the United States costs almost $9,000 ("Great News for the Dead"), I want to get the most for my money. Thanks to Dad, who set up my lifelong insurance plan, I have a policy that should cover not only the cremation and memorial celebration, but extra costs like postage and handling my remains to send some of my ashes to Indiana. I also want a headstone that, like a giant X, marks the spot where my remains will remain. Thanks to my sometimes taking on two part-time jobs in addition to my full-time employment early in my career, my trust should have enough money to cover more than the estimated $9,000 for my cremation and interment or ash distribution. *The Economist* article teasingly suggests that the key questions for family members overseeing post-death rites are "burn or bury?" (I want both!) and "check or card?" (either will work when the money comes from my insurance policy or my trust account). If my preparations go according to plan, the trust's executor will know how to answer any undertaker's questions and have the means to make my wishes come true.

My decisions regarding what I cheerfully refer to as "disposing of the body," likely a result of too many Sherlock Holmes stories, and my memorial celebration are, like many parts of my philosophy and lifestyle, a hodgepodge. They are based on my early religious experiences and later rituals that I encountered through popular culture or travel. My earliest memories of Protestant funerals, often in small rural Indiana communities, involve country church services and a gathering of friends and family after the gravesite visit. When I was a child, I often accompanied Mom and Mom-Ma Margie to funerals or cemeteries. We dressed solemnly for the service, said our goodbyes at the open coffin, sang hymns, prayed, listened to a minister talk about the deceased's life and afterlife, and rode in a long procession of cars to the cemetery for a shorter service before the coffin was lowered into the grave. Afterward, if Mom-Ma Margie or Mom knew the recently departed well, we stopped by the deceased's or a relative's house to share food and talk quietly. When I was five or six, I could never run or play at these events or, in fact, do anything to muss my starched-petticoat dress or black patent-leather shoes. I quietly nibbled a cookie or sandwich and listened to sad grownups whisper. Sometimes I was called forth to be introduced and commented upon before going away again to sit quietly. By the time I was in my mid-teens, I was expected to make small talk with strangers who knew my relatives in another place or time. What was more difficult was crying on command. Although I felt sorrowful when a loved one died, I had learned by the time I was seven or eight to suck up any negative emotions and not cause a fuss. Mom sometimes told me that the neighbors (or teachers or other family members) would wonder what was wrong with me—or with my parents' parenting—if I cried where others could see. At school, unable to kick or hit back at bullies, who only attacked harder if I tried, I finally learned to avoid confrontations and refuse to admit pain. However, when I couldn't produce an appropriate volume of tears during a funeral, Mom worriedly asked why I couldn't cry. Fortunately, as an adult I had become much better at comforting others, and so I could at least be useful at funeral home viewings, funeral services, and after-funeral gatherings. Being outwardly unemotional also prepared me to deliver appropriately memorable eulogies at Dad's, Mom's, and Bart's services. Just in case my memorial involves a lot of weepers who might choke up eulogizing me (and also because I like to control details and am a planner), I wrote my own obituary that can double as a handy eulogy. Also, I frequently toy with the idea of making a farewell video that says exactly what I would want others to say about me. My friends, however, have assured me that this might be kind of creepy.

Just as memorable as the funerals during my childhood was the ritual after-funeral gathering—and its food. When Mom-Ma Margie died in the late 1980s, everyone associated with the mourners dropped off food at her tiny house on Chestnut Street in Evansville. My favorite dish was sent by Genie's mother, gentle, thoughtful Marie Horn. She instructed Genie to drop off a bowl of strawberries packed in sugar, which, by the time we returned to Mom-Ma's house from the funeral, had created a sweet bowl of berries swimming in juicy splendor.

When Dad died, neighbors and a representative from the United Methodist Church in Leesburg, Florida, brought covered dishes of meats and vegetables, some in casseroles. The counter in Mom's kitchen supported a crowd of pies—cherry, apple, blueberry, coconut cream, lemon, pecan, peanut butter. As recent retirees and new Florida transplants, my parents didn't have many friends locally, but a few people with whom Dad had worked at Western-Southern Life attended his Florida funeral. (Dad had two funerals—one in Florida, primarily so his father could attend—and one in Indiana, where he was buried.)

Since my paternal grandmother died and my grandfather found himself lonely and unsure how to live alone, I had seen little of him. One day Pop-Pa sold his house and everything in it to a man who came to the door, asking if he would sell. This decision didn't sit well with Dad, in particular—the piano and china Mom-Ma Polly promised me, in addition to Dad's childhood memorabilia and duck calls, were part of the sentimental loss to that sale. Within a few months, Pop-Pa remarried and, before long, moved from Indiana to Florida to be near his new wife's daughter's family. Thus, my grandfather and his newly acquired stepson drove from Bradenton to Leesburg for the funeral. As expected, they came to my parents' house on the lake, not so much to mourn collectively but, as I later learned, mostly to check on procedures to cash in the insurance policy Dad had taken out for Pop-Pa more than 40 years earlier. (I don't mean to seem callous, but, when I called Pop-Pa to tell him that Dad was gone, his wife answered the phone and only let me talk to my grandfather after I angrily told her that I thought he might like to know his son had died. Dad was an only child, and I really do believe Pop-Pa grieved for him. He just sometimes had a strange way of showing his love or concern.) After sharing the post-funeral meal, Pop-Pa took Bart for a little walk out in the backyard where it was quieter. They strolled to the end of the pier on the lake—truly an unfortunate place for Pop-Pa to inquire about the life insurance policy. Bart almost pushed his grandfather into the alligator-infested water. Red-faced, Bart held his temper long enough to storm into the house. This was the last time either of us saw our grandfather. Although most after-funeral meals are quiet affairs, occasionally there is enough entertainment to fuel gossip for years.

To help me decide whether I wanted to break further from the "meal back at the house" tradition and the solemnity of the typical Protestant funeral, I studied other cultures' traditions regarding death. As a TED Ideas article notes, funeral practices and memorial celebrations vary widely by culture. Author Kate Torgovnick May explained the New Orleans jazz funeral, for example, as well as such diverse rituals as Ghana's "fantasy coffins" representing something the deceased loved in life or South Korean burial beads made from the compressed ashes of the deceased. Emotionally, I connect with these types of public mourning and celebrations of life, although they are far from my upbringing.

However, I have at least witnessed one of these celebrations of the deceased's life. One evening, as a group of friends and I celebrated arriving in New Orleans by enjoying dinner outdoors at the Palace Café on Canal Street, we heard the whoop of a police siren and saw flashing lights of cars clearing the way for a jazz funeral of a high-ranking public official. Heedless of politeness (or the delicious crab cheesecake), I bolted from the table and ran to the corner to watch the funeral cortege cross Canal and continue down Chartres. Not only did mournful notes break into buoyant brass as mourners danced down the street, but the horse-drawn black hearse allowed those of us crowded onto the sidewalk a clear view of the deceased lying in state. This ritual is not part of my culture, but I love the joy of celebrating life, as well as a life, in the midst of sorrow. Taking this sentiment to guide me, I began planning death rituals unique to me but that hint at my cultural past. More important, they represent the life I lived and the celebration instead of sorrow I want to encourage upon my passing.

What might seem even weirder than a personalized cultural hodge-podge is my enjoyment of the planning process. The longer I lived post-terminal diagnosis, the more I appreciated being able to infuse my personality into the business of death: writing my obituary, making my wishes known about a small memorial service, and disposing of my remains. Being a control freak has its perks when it comes to notifying the public of my death and planning a celebration of me.

Some ideas for these tasks come from my travels or popular culture. For example, during a tour of Christiansfeld, a Moravian community and UNESCO World Heritage site in Denmark, the guide explained a Moravian tradition of writing a letter to the community near the end of one's lifetime. Upon the writer's death, the letter is read during the funeral ceremony. Whereas the original purpose of these letters may have involved a plea for forgiveness or spoken to one's values upheld in life, more recent letters have verged on leaving a final good impression or cementing one's legacy as a successful member of the community.

Three years before my trip to Denmark, Bart wrote a farewell editorial to his colleagues at work. As a communications specialist, he often wrote articles for websites or newsletters. Throughout his career as a journalist or corporate communications writer/editor, he had published plenty of news articles, reports, and editorials; at home, he wrote novels and stories. Thus, for both of us, writing became the preferred way to communicate our feelings, thanks, and even humor as we say goodbye. Bart's editorial was shared with co-workers after his death, but it also served as a self-eulogy to be shared with others online.

Keeping Bart and the Danish Moravian community in mind, I chose to write a series of letters—personalized farewells to individual friends or family members. However, I also took charge of writing my own obituary to send to the *Evansville Courier-Press* in my old hometown and to the *Daytona Beach News-Journal*. Both forms of documentation will note my passing to friends, family, former colleagues, and associates in my birthplace and my most recent workplace. Here is my personalized obituary, written for accuracy and expediency, so that this is one less task for anyone to do when I am dead.

> Lynnette Raye Porter, originally from Evansville, Indiana, but most recently from Ormond Beach, Florida, died _____. [Although one psychic has told me that, for a fee, she can tell me the date of my death, (1) I am skeptical that she knows, and I likely won't be able to get a refund if she is wrong, and (2) I really don't want to know. It is bad enough for my oncologist and me to guess.] Lynnette was the daughter of Charles Raymond (Ray) and Doris James (Jimmie) Porter and the sister of Bartley Alan Porter, all who preceded her in death. She leaves behind her sister-in-law, Nancy Porter; niece, Heather Porter; great-nephew, Levi Williams; and great-niece, Ava Williams, as well as many cousins and friends. Lynnette was a 1975 graduate of Harrison High School in Evansville and earned her M.A. in technical writing (1983) and Ph.D. in English, rhetoric, composition, Victorian literature, and technical communication (1989) from Bowling Green State University in Ohio. She was tenured at the University of Findlay in Ohio and Embry-Riddle Aeronautical University in Daytona Beach, Florida, where she attained the rank of Professor. In addition, she worked as a technical writer, trainer, and editor and was a Fellow in the Society for Technical Communication. During her long career, she wrote or co-authored 21 books [I am optimistic about two books in progress], most about popular culture; was a columnist and contributing editor to online magazine *PopMatters*; and served as editor of the Popular Culture Association in the South's journal, *Studies in Popular Culture*. She loved to travel, in particular, throughout New Zealand, Canada, Iceland, Scotland, and Wales. A memorial service will be held _____ on _____.

In my handy "manual for Lynnette's afterdeath" (once a technical writer, always a technical writer), I even listed the cost and place to email this obituary to two newspapers representing my past and present affiliations. Although I can't guarantee that the eulogy will appear online or in print, I hope that my careful planning will lead to one final publication.

Not only do I want people to read this writer's words about herself, but I would like for my memorial service to allow reflection on television or film dialogue or passages from novels that reflect my philosophy. For example, lines such as these might be shared during a dramatic reading at my memorial service or through an online death announcement:

In one of my all-time favorite *Doctor Who* episodes, "School Reunion," the Tenth Doctor (David Tennant) agrees with the wisdom of former companion Sarah Jane Smith (Elisabeth Sladen, who, I note, but do not limit her significance to her medical history, also died of cancer), when she discussed the aftermath of their shared time in the TARDIS: "The universe has to move forward. Pain and loss, they define us as much as happiness or love.... Everything has its time. And everything ends."

In "The Lazarus Experiment," the Tenth Doctor adds to my philosophy by espousing part of his own, that "some people live more in twenty years than others do in eighty. It's not the time that matters, it's the person."

Finally, in another one of my all-time favorites, the Vincent van Gogh episode entitled "Vincent and the Doctor," the Eleventh Doctor (Matt Smith) explains to the troubled artist, "The way I see it, every life is a pile of good things and ... bad things. The good things don't always soften the bad things, but vice versa, the bad things don't necessarily spoil the good things or make them unimportant" ["30 Pieces of Wisdom from Doctor Who"].

Perhaps, after reading or hearing these words of wisdom provided by a Doctor (and his traveling companions) that I implicitly trust and whose advice I willingly follow, those attending my memorial—or, as I prefer to think of it, a party to celebrate my life and the love among us—can ponder the relevance of some of my favorite lines to my life. (Feel free to discuss amongst yourselves.)

I hope that part of my legacy is my enjoyment of life. Despite the cancer, I have lived my life to the fullest and enjoyed far more days than the number I have been in pain or sadness. Whereas a cancer diagnosis often is only considered as one of the "bad things" that the Eleventh Doctor notes, this disease also has made me more aware of what life means and how to enjoy it and the power and strength of love between my friends and family and me. However, I am also grateful for the important human connection and moments of grace from a casual encounter with a student or a stranger, for example. Although I don't wish to be remembered only as someone who had cancer (or died from it), I am aware that having cancer is one of the most important things to ever happen to me. For one, it has made me cognizant of the business of dying I need to take care of, as well as my quirky way of taking care of business.

Just as emotionally fulfilling and self-aggrandizing as writing about myself for an obituary or a eulogy and suggesting "readings" for my memorial service is choosing the music to play at a gathering that could be held in my condo (once someone dusts the furniture and mops the kitchen floor), at a friend's home, or even beachside at a venue rented for a few hours. The event should be held a week or more after my death to allow anyone traveling from out of state to arrive—and possibly spend a few days at the Orlando theme parks or along a Florida beach while they're in town. I would like a toast to be made in my honor and for friends and family to take turns telling stories or sharing memories, just as Nancy did for Bart. In the background, my final playlist should set the mood for the commemoration of my life and the likely reunion of family members who have not seen each other since the last funeral or memorial brought them together.

I thoroughly enjoyed going through my favorite death-themed songs to choose my Top 10 playlist for my memorial. These are my selections in the order in which they should be played:

"Another One Bites the Dust"—Queen
"Dust in the Wind"—Kansas
"Don't Fear the Reaper"—Blue Öyster Cult
"Candle in the Wind"—Elton John
"Who Wants to Live Forever?"—Queen
"Knockin' on Heaven's Door"—Bob Dylan
"Angel"—Sarah McLachlan
"The Impossible Dream"—Scott Bakula version from *Quantum Leap*
"Turn Turn Turn"—The Byrds
"The Last Goodbye"—Billy Boyd, *The Hobbit: The Battle of the Five Armies*

Each one has a special meaning, representing a specific time in my life or a memory of the situations in which I enjoyed those songs.

The irreverent choice is Queen, especially "Another One Bites the Dust." "Knockin' on Heaven's Door" is probably a rude choice. During my weekend-long celebration of my Lifetime Achievement Award as a researcher/writer at Embry-Riddle Aeronautical University, an honor which had been bestowed during the Humanities and Communication Department's annual spring dinner in 2018, I enjoyed sitting outdoors to hear The Shores' guitarist. When he began the first notes of "Knockin' on Heaven's Door," I queried whether any of my friends had requested or dedicated the song to me. Needless to say, those around me who hadn't had a second rum runner didn't find my comment humorous. Still, the song seems appropriate for a final send-off—and maybe everyone surrounding my urn will be enjoying rum runners or a decent Scotch to help them applaud my selection.

Most of my musical choices reflect my fandoms and love of popular culture interwoven with travel experiences. I associate "Who Wants to Live Forever?" with the television series *Highlander* and hunky immortals Duncan MacLeod (Adrian Paul) and Methos (Peter Wingfield, who was a fine conversationalist and photo op good sport at a Chicago fan conference I attended in 2008). "Candle in the Wind" reminds me of listening to Elton John while waiting for a friend to finish an out-of-state job interview and then feeling out of place during a decidedly unromantic Valentine's Day dinner in a strange town. Perhaps that's not the best memory, because it represents an awkward occasion, but that trip gave me the opportunity to reunite with Elton John music after a long hiatus.

"Angel" reflects my 1990s infatuation with Sarah McLachlan: I traveled the Midwest to follow at least three of her Lilith Fair concerts in three different cities for each of the festival's three years during the late '90s. I faithfully bought each Sarah McLachlan CD at the big HMV on Yonge Street during my frequent visits to Toronto, and I embraced her as part of my Paul Gross/*Due South* infatuation. (Some of her early songs were part of the television series' soundtrack.) "Angel" also was a song Bart and I selected as the sole secular song played at Mom's funeral.

Like "Angel," "The Impossible Dream" has a convoluted association with my life. One of my favorite *Quantum Leap* episodes, "Catch a Falling Star—May 21, 1979," summarizes my fannish love for series star Scott Bakula, who sings "The Impossible Dream" as part of this *Man of La Mancha*-themed episode. In 1996, I flew to Los Angeles to see him perform twice (with Carol Burnett) at the Hollywood Bowl. Later that year, I again flew to LA to attend a Leapers' convention (and see Bakula). In 2011 I chatted with Bakula during a San Diego ComicCon/Nerd Herd presentation and post-discussion meet-and-greet. The fact that one of my favorite actors sang one of my favorite songs from one of my first-favorite musicals makes "The Impossible Dream" an especially meaningful choice.

Finally, "The Last Goodbye" is the result of another favored fan crush. Billy Boyd—Pippin in the *Lord of the Rings* films—wrote the music and lyrics to the end-credit song to the final film in Peter Jackson's *Hobbit* trilogy. Not only did I meet Boyd several times when I was an academic speaker at *Lord of the Rings* fan conventions in the United States and U.K. during the mid–2000s, but my spiritual home is New Zealand, where the *Lord of the Rings* and *Hobbit* movies were filmed. In 2012, I attended the Wellington festivities surrounding the first *Hobbit* film's New Zealand premiere (and, at a local bookshop, enjoyed signing copies of one of my hobbit-themed books). In addition, for decades Merry Brandybuck and Pippin Took have been my favorite hobbit characters. A song written by "Pippin" Boyd, especially one that references Tolkien's characters and closed the Made in New Zealand film trilogies that had been the focus of my research and travel activities for nearly a decade, is a must-have on the playlist. The lyrics to Boyd's song presumably refer to Bilbo saying farewell at the end of his long life's journey, but the song also represented Jackson and company's farewell to their devoted audiences at the end of both the *Lord of the Rings* trilogy and the subsequent *Hobbit* trilogy. For me, this last song in my memorial playlist summarizes my love of this fandom, my memories of tours and sabbaticals all over New Zealand, and my final farewell to my loved ones. This selection is a very "me" way to have the last word and to guarantee that there will not be a dry eye in my house, or wherever my memorial toast and background playlist celebrate my life. I would write that my ears probably will burn as a result of everyone talking about my strange choices in celebrating the recently deceased me, but, by then, my ears should already have been incinerated during cremation.

I also have grand plans for my body's fiery send-off. If possible, I prefer a Viking-style pyre pushed off Ormond Beach and ignited by an arrow shot from shore. My inspiration is King Arthur's fire-at-sea funeral portrayed in the final moments of *First Knight* (1995). Not only do I enjoy a good Camelot film—or even a not-so-good one like *First Knight*—but Arthur's pagan immolation increased my critical estimation of the film. However, the likelihood of getting the necessary paperwork to fulfill this fantasy post-death is even less than the hope that all my legal wrangling and planning will be smoothly executed after my death. Thus, as somewhat of a compromise, I request that half of my cremated remains be spread along Ormond Beach and within the waves so that I can be both part of the landscape I love and an eternal global sea traveler. I also want to be piped to my bon voyage by a Scottish bagpiper wearing a tartan, a nod to my Scottish ancestry. The other half of my ashes should be sent to Indiana to be buried next to my parents; I want a headstone to immortalize the dates of my life. In this way, I strive one final time to please my parents and follow their wishes that I be buried in the family plot. There is nothing better than trying to please everyone with the funereal celebrations. At least I won't hear any complaints.

CHAPTER 7

Who Am I?

A variation to the lyrics of The Who's "Who Are You" has lead vocalist Roger Daltrey (as the voice of Pete Townshend, whose experiences led to his writing this song) looking in the mirror, at times even posing, as he ponders who he is and how far he has come (for better or, as the song posits, more likely for worse) since he first became a musician. Comparing who he has become with who he was is not always a positive revelation. The lyric that most fans likely recall, however, is the insistently repeated title question, followed by a hoot-owl chorus of "who"s. In the immediate aftermath of my terminal diagnosis, I metaphorically looked in the mirror many times and, months afterward, continue to ponder my identity. Who am I? Do I have a new identity simply as a result of having cancer, or has my identity changed with the arrival of Stage 4? Is the body I present to the world a variation or a betrayal of my most recent incarnation as a fan/scholar, a nurturing auntie, a mentor to colleagues, a close friend? Has cancer created a new me, or am I an evolution of what I have been? Am I still entitled to be part of the human family, or have I become more "other"?

In a review of the *Who Are You* album, *Rolling Stone* declared that Daltrey's delivery emphasizes uncertainty: "'I really want to know!' Daltrey shouts back [in answer to the title question, and he] is desperate, sure of nothing" (Marcus). I began my cancer journey feeling desperate, but, as I have analyzed the less-than-steadily-linear progression of the disease and my musings about my life, I found that I really want to know who I am. Through new experiences as mundane as riding an inner tube down a resort's lazy river, getting a Himalayan salt stone massage, or tasting dried haddock, I learn more about myself: my likes and dislikes, my willingness to try something just for the experience, my quest for *more*. I must prioritize how I spend time and money, and my choices often surprise me about what I really think or want.

I have no scientific evidence that my ponderings or personal experiments are accurate in assessing who I am, and thus, in a sense, I am sure of nothing. However, my limited little out-of-body experiences surrounding surgeries or, during a brief but memorable time during chemo when I couldn't breathe and only Jen's timely intervention resulted in my being revived with a burst of pure oxygen, lead me to conclude, as Daltrey does in his memoir, that the transition from life to death may be peaceful and nothing to fear. In Daltrey's near-death experience, he saw no white light at the end of a tunnel but revisited his life and felt reassured that he had left behind no unfinished business—his loved ones were looked after. In my less dramatic possible-last-moments, I, too, felt peace and security in the knowledge that I had done as much as possible, especially near the end, to make amends or help out in little ways. In the ensuing months after my terminal diagnosis, I sometimes awakened because I briefly stopped breathing. Aware of gasping and feeling almost as if in a dream, I struggled to get air and heard my breath rattle in my chest. Each time I awoke in distress, I was able to sit up or roll onto my side and, heart pounding, breathe regularly once again. I accept that someday I may not be able to awaken or breathe—but that possible way of dying seems only momentarily frightening. Although I can prove nothing definitively about death based on these few instances of my brain briefly being deprived of oxygen, I don't fear the transition from life to death but feel satisfied and grateful for the life I have been able to lead.

What I have learned thus far from my identity quest is that I am now truly a paradox. I don't desire to be defined by my disease but persist in defining myself by what I can and can't do because of it. I live and rejoice in each day's liveliness but am aware that I am temporally and medically that much closer to death. I am enjoying life more than I ever have but am cognizant of a greater sadness in seeing that life end.

Lately I compare myself to the theoretical Schrödinger's cat. A *New Scientist* article summarizes Erwin Schrödinger's thought experiment that could demonstrate the absurdity of the Copenhagen interpretation of quantum theory, which permits things to be two ways at once. As the *Washington Post* describes this interpretation, it "suggested that particles existed in all possible states (different positions, energies or speeds) until they were observed, at which point they collapsed into one set state" (Feltman). Schrödinger planned his experiment to show that this interpretation is faulty when larger things, such as a cat, are involved. The simple version of his thought experiment's design is this: "you take a cat and stick it in a box rigged up with a radioactive atom, a hammer and a vial of poisonous gas. The atom decays, and this triggers the hammer to fall and break the vial, suffocating the cat. Or not." Even in science, with its laws and frequent predictability, not everything is certain. For example, "radioactive decays are random processes described by quantum theory, so we can't say when one will happen. And quantum theory strongly suggests that before you observe or measure an object, it exists in a 'superposition' of all its possible states. Before we open the box, the atom is both decayed and undecayed—and the cat both dead and alive" (Amit).

Perhaps another, far less scientific way to think of being dead and undead at the same time is to recall a pivotal scene from *Star Trek II: The Wrath of Khan* (1982), or the "Spock in a box" conundrum, based on dialogue from Montgomery Scott (James Doohan). When Spock (Leonard Nimoy) enters a radioactive chamber to get the *Enterprise* back online so the crew can get away from (the wrath of) Khan (Ricardo Montalban), Admiral James T. Kirk's (William Shatner) mortal enemy, he immediately becomes saturated with deadly radioactivity. Horrified to learn what his First Officer and close friend has done to save the ship, Kirk moves to open the chamber to get Spock out. Scotty helps hold back the Admiral, telling him that Spock is "dead already." Yet, dead/alive Spock still has a few minutes for a heart-to-heart with Kirk before succumbing to the deadly radiation. During that scene, Spock is apparently Schrödinger's cat. That is, Spock is simultaneously both alive and dead until Kirk "observes" him in the clear-walled enclosure and, voilà, "the whole dead-and-alive-until-proven-otherwise-and-then-suddenly-you're-either-dead-or-alive thing" (Feltman) occurs. In Spock's case, he is dead—at least until the next film in the series.

Although I can't count on a sequel or a franchise reboot to bring me back, I can relate to Spock in this scene and Schrödinger's cat in the box. In all our cases, we have been exposed to radiation and are "poisoned" by something deadly. At least theoretically, we can be both alive and dead for some period of time. Whereas a terminal diagnosis and short prognosis have shifted my focus from death as something abstract in the far future to a process requiring more immediate attention, I also must remember that, as of this moment, I am living with cancer, not only dying as a result of it. It is the *knowing* (the "observation" stage) that tips the balance into one state or another. I now know that my body is dying. Even though I think positively and try to focus on what is happening now, rather than agonize over what may or will happen, I have observed the scans of my body and heard professional opinions about what those scans mean. I am getting ever closer to the stage when the cat's box is going to be opened or Spock presses his hand against the glass in a Vulcan salute and, with his final words, commands Kirk to "live long and prosper."

I am a consistent dichotomy, a study in oppositions. I am cancerous tumors and healthy cells. I am terminally ill and feeling healthier than I have in five years. (My oncologist says the only thing wrong with me is cancer.) I am elderly in years but childlike in gratitude and joy. I am less attractive physically to others but more at peace with the way I present myself to the world. I am more aware of my body but trying harder to ignore random splashes of pain and increasing instances when I must pause to catch my breath. I don't wish to be pigeonholed as a terminally ill person, a dying woman, a cancerous being. Yet, I also am forthright about my diagnosis and prognosis and choose to spend a great deal of time during my last months writing a book about being cancerous. Such is the paradox of my being terminally ill with metastatic cancer.

Ironically, a little book entitled *Tumor* helped clarify my self-definition and struggle with my current or persistent physical identity. As author Anna Leahy notes, "*cancer* and *tumor* are part of the social conversation of who we are" (50), as she documents the secrecy and silence historically surrounding a cancer diagnosis. Even today, and despite my determination to be open in answering others' questions about my health, cancer is not the most important part of my life. Until my physical appearance reveals that I am very ill, my niece's children, my close friends' children, and the majority of my cousins aren't aware that I have cancer (or, in some cases, that my cancer has returned after surgery and chemo). Until my physical body makes my condition obvious to anyone who sees me, I look "normal" and avoid being publicly associated with cancer. I prefer to keep others innocent of the knowledge of my prognosis, largely because the word *cancer* probably (and, in my case, quite accurately) is perceived as a death sentence.

Death is still a fearsome, abstract concept to the children in my life, and I don't want to cause them anxiety about what is going to happen to me or, someday, to their loved ones and themselves. As my dying becomes more obvious and active, I hope I will be able to explain what is happening to me and to answer their questions about my experience with dying. However, more important, I hope that through our shared time while I was and while I look healthy—at Disney World, on the beach, at school events, at home during holidays and birthday parties—they will remember that, for many months longer than expected, I was playful, thoughtful, funny, exasperated, caring, cautionary, determined, and demonstrative—like I always had been around them. "Dying," for me, is a lengthier process than anticipated after a terminal diagnosis but leads to a shorter number of years than I hoped to share with them. Who I am and should remain to them is Aunt Lynnette or Auntie Nette, not a fearsome dying creature because of the word *cancer*.

In the case of my cousins who seldom hear from me outside of annual Christmas cards or more frequent Facebook posts, I don't wish pity, and, unfortunately and perhaps unfairly, that response is what I expect to receive. (Well, I hope no one cheers when they hear about my diagnosis or death!) To date, I haven't announced my illness via social media. I am afraid that, if my prognosis becomes widespread common knowledge, I will automatically become "other" simply because of some cells or tumors in my body. My diagnosis may limit my Facebook friends' perception of me to "someone who died of cancer," as if other details of my life aren't equally or more memorable or significant. I don't want to cause sorrow—and if someone can hear of my cancer diagnosis, acknowledge it, and let us both get on with our lives as normally as possible, that's all I want. It is not, however, what I expect will occur.

In part, my expectations are derived from the common language most Americans use to describe cancer. I admit that I am part of the problem of using language that separates the cancer (or in my case, my perception of *body*) from the rest of the person (my perception of *mind* or *spirit*). Although I very much believe that mind/body/spirit is and should be realized as a whole, as one, I struggle with this part of my identity when organs physically do not perform the way they are meant to or when physiological damage (i.e., the "new normal" post-disease progression or post-surgeries) is difficult to reconcile with my physical self-image. Leahy explains that language such as a *fight* or a *battle* with cancer, in which cancer is envisioned as an *invader* or an *enemy* and therefore is something to *beat*, "dismisses the biological fact that the tumor is part of and is made out of one's own body" (51). I accept that Leahy is correct, but "love me, love my tumors" is still difficult.

If a cancer patient isn't a warrior fighting cancer, Leahy asks, is that patient somehow less than expected, or just less a person, if she or he is angry, frightened, depressed, or passive? After all, cancer does take a lot out of a person—literally (through tumor or organ removal, through exhaustion) and figuratively (through emotional swings). Just as I am trying to do with my memoir, so Leahy strives to do with her book— we both look for ways to dispel stigmas surrounding cancer and to realistically depict what is becoming a common cultural experience: having cancer or knowing someone who does. Leahy recognizes, as do I, that the common assumption that "a passive, impotent cancer patient who is angry about his or her fate is a far less appealing sight (and site) than a brave, upbeat go-getter who helps those around him deal with the situation with courage and warmth" (54). Yet, that's not why I embrace my joy at every sunrise and feel gratitude every night. Sometimes I wonder if my friends and family, some who call me their "light" or "sunshine," trust my gratitude as genuine, or if they think that I'm only successfully playing the role of a grateful woman.

Some people who run into me or have come into my office are tense if the conversation turns to my health. They may be unaware of their suddenly stiffened spine or slight step back; they often avert their eyes by looking down or to the side. Their voice may become quieter or their pitch drop as they ask how I'm feeling. In short, their demeanor projects seriousness and uncertainty. Such was the case as I stood waiting for an elevator in the university's student union one afternoon, when two colleagues I hadn't seen for months suddenly recognized me as they walked toward the lift. The difference in their approach couldn't have been more obvious, despite the fact that I knew both of them equally. We had been friendly at university receptions and during classroom presentations, but we weren't close friends. One woman (I'll dub her Ms. Shy) hung back, letting her co-worker take the lead physically and socially. She glanced down and away while her widely smiling colleague (I'll call her Ms. Gregarious) walked right up into my personal space to greet me and asked about my health, quietly confiding that she'd heard from a friend in my department that my cancer had returned. She wasn't squeamish about asking about cancer but thoughtfully lowered her voice so as not to broadcast my prognosis to everyone in the hallway. Ms. Gregarious maintained eye contact, nodded thoughtfully when I assured her that I was still feeling well, and spontaneously hugged me at that good news. At that point, Ms. Shy came closer to say hello and join the conversation. From reading nonverbal cues (which sometimes aren't as obvious as they are in this example), I know that some people are relieved because I'm meeting their expectations of the courageous cancer fighter rather than being "depressing" when we talk.

When I'm being honest about the state of my body, I worry that I'm inadvertently cruel to the very people I want to spare pain. After the October 2018 visit to my oncologist, who pointed out that my lung tumors had grown minimally in the past six months and declared that "on a scale of 10, with 10 being you're cured, this news is a 9," I cheerfully called friends or family around the country to share the good news. Because I was so bubbly and announced, "I have good news I want to tell you!" as soon as the phone was answered, more than once my enthusiasm misled people into the false conclusion that my cancer had gone away or the diagnosis was wrong. "I knew they were wrong!" was often the immediate response, leading to an awkward pause before I had to admit that I am still terminally ill, although my prognosis has been prolonged. A dejected "oh" precedes a lengthier silence and the inevitably flat-toned "I thought you had really good news." What is excellent news to me can still be devastating in its implications for those I love.

Throughout my life I have interpreted others' negative or painful emotional responses as somehow being "all my fault" and tried very hard not to cause anyone a problem. However, that deep-rooted tendency doesn't negate my current enjoyment of life. I may not be actively embroiled in fighting cancer, but I am fortunate to continue actively living my life—going to work, visiting loved ones, traveling. At the opposite end of the courageous warrior continuum is the passive cancer patient, or, as some family members think of it, someone who has given up.

Whereas some hang onto the image of me heroically fighting to defeat cancer, others believe that I have become a prisoner of war, a victim and soon-to-be casualty of a lost battle. Doing *something* more obviously battle oriented—whether eating a carefully proscribed diet, taking chemo, or going somewhere for alternative treatments—would mean, to them, that I am fighting for my life. Just as I am not trying to be a fighter—I just *am*, living each day the best way I can—so am I not a loser or a victim just because I am not actively seeking a cure.

Others' interpretations of life with cancer or, more specifically, my life with cancer may lead to biases or comments about what a cancer patient should or should not be able to do, what someone with a terminal diagnosis should or should not do to prolong life, even whether someone with cancer is mentally competent once the body deteriorates. I have run into many well-meaning people, as well as some who have been rude or judgmental, who share their ideas about what I should do next. Many lyrics in the mainstream version of The Who's "Who Are You" emphasize the word *you*, questioning who these people around the rock star are and why or if they should influence the singer. I also ask "Who are *you*?" when I determine who among my inner circle should be allowed to advise me and try to persuade me to change my mind. I ask the same question when I consider how much influence relative strangers, whether the proverbial man on the street or a medical professional, should have over my choices and decisions. I don't claim to know much scientifically about cancer in general or colorectal cancer specifically. Therefore, I invite the people I trust to tell me their suggestions or ideas that can have an impact on my life. However, it is my life, and death, and, ultimately, the decisions about the ways I respond to my diagnosis and prognosis are my responsibility.

As Leahy notes, that was not always the case and still is not in many cultures; doctors or family members who want to shield someone with cancer from that news in order to spare them fear and possibly to extend their lifespan simply do not reveal the prognosis to the patient. Cancer has been and often remains stigmatized; it is a whispered word or a pitying glance. Most people have opinions and ideas about cancer—and therefore people with cancer—and are willing to share them, for better or worse. It is up to those with cancer to ask "Who are *you*?" in their lives and how much credence will be given to which opinions and ideas or, indeed, which people. Even out of context, The Who's popular lyrics can invite some important self-searching and consideration of which people are allowed a say in the way one's life is led or end of life takes place.

Unfortunately, my and many others' physical identity is based on societal expectations and definitions of physical perfection that somehow have become equated with a person's worth. Not only may my physical identity revolve around what my body can or cannot do or what others expect it to do or not do because of cancer, but the attractiveness of that body forms a huge part of the way I am categorized as desirable. Just as people aren't as thrilled to be around a depressed or angry cancer patient, so, too, are they not as compelled to be near a prematurely aged or withered body or one connected to drips or monitors.

In many Western societies, especially those heavily influenced by American images of beauty as purveyed through advertisements, films, and television series, I am identified as "other" because of my failure to meet expectations of beauty. Many studies "indicate that the standard of beauty widely presented on television, movies, and video games is having a powerful effect on adolescents. This effect reinforces low self-esteem that can lead to risky behavior [sic] such as excessive dieting" (Vitelli). I posit that adolescents and young adults are not the only ones who base their self-identity or feelings of self-worth on media depictions of beauty; basing my identity on a societal definition of beauty has been a problem throughout my life.

In my mid–20s to early 30s, my physical self-identity primarily reflected the opinions of those closest to me—including but not limited to family, fellow grad students, employers, and love interests. I starved myself, worked out to Jane Fonda videos, attended Jazzercise classes, and carefully coiffed and dressed myself to reflect the desired image of a successful professional woman. I worked hard and, for a time, succeeded in meeting a Midwest-filtered version of California-esque sexual and professional attractiveness.

In my late post-menopausal 50s, I still recognized the high bar of attractiveness (i.e., tall, thin, young, clear complexioned, straight white toothed) that women are expected to meet, but I already was gazing at it from far below as I struggled to inconspicuously limbo beneath it and quietly enter my 60s. (How low would I go?) I wasn't even comforted by the fact that the film stars to whom students or potential or actual lovers flatteringly compared me in my 20s—Faye Dunaway, Candace Bergen, Kathleen Turner (in *Body Heat* [1981], no less!)—also had gained weight and facial lines (or facelifts). I accepted that I would never have a body like Helen Mirren's at 22 or 72.

However, my initial cancer diagnosis made any hope or desire to achieve an acceptable level of attractiveness vanish. My rectal surgery resulted in an ileostomy for eight months. Although many people do well with an ileostomy, I often had problems ranging from a lengthy inability to find an appliance that would fit and not leak, a leaky bag that left my abdomen with "acid" burns from liquid waste, and baggy eyes from lack of sleep because I had to empty the bag every hour or two. Stretch pants were my best fashion option because they accommodated the bag as it expanded. Surgery gave me a longer life—for which I am grateful, even if the cancer likely had already metastasized by the time the rectal tumor was removed; those traveling cancer cells just hadn't shown up on scans yet and would prove to be resistant to chemo. However, surgery also gave me scars and an unevenly shaped lower body. My skin and blood vessels are not as elastic post-chemotherapy, and cancer has increased the rate at which I age.

Post-ileostomy reversal, as I have described in probably too much detail throughout this book, has decreased the likelihood that I will ever be considered an "attractive" companion. I wear not only an adult diaper (or sometimes two) but plastic pants beneath my clothes, and sometimes even those barriers don't stop leaks when my digestive system kicks into high gear. Changes in hormones, not only because of menopause but from the removal of an ovary during cancer surgery, helped thicken my waistline and add a roll of flab. Of course, I can't passively blame treatments or surgeries for everything about my appearance. When I took chemotherapy, I could eat anything I wanted and not gain weight. Giving up the luxury of highly caloric meals at the end of chemo has been difficult, and my terminal diagnosis further made dieting unappealing. During the months when I feared that another DVT or PE might kill me before the cancer could, I gave up even gentle yoga and long walks on the beach. I haven't given in to looking older, fatter, and wrinklier, but I pay more attention to enjoying what I can eat or drink than counting calories. Exercise includes those long beach walks again, but some days I prefer to take a book to the beach or watch the waves. I take care to apply makeup and dress stylishly for my body size and type. Despite those actions, I know that I am "other" from the societal conception of a beautiful woman, even one of "advanced age."

Cancer marks people as the disease progresses and forces a "dead" person to recognize physical changes that become increasingly evident to everyone. Identifying oneself mostly by body image can be traumatic when that body ages and dies. Even accepting that cancer is part of my body may not ease the distress of physical discomfort or the psychological pain at realizing that I do not look like I used to, still want to, or am expected to in order to be socially acceptable. What is worse is that I may no longer be able to do everyday tasks—grocery shopping, doing the laundry, taking out the trash, driving—or, when I do them, I lurch along, stop frequently, turn red in the face, or gasp for air. Walking up stairs is becoming more of a chore, and I can't avoid the realization that, just as during my chemo treatments, I may soon be unable to trot up the stairs with a load of laundry—or even haltingly take a step on flat ground. Who *are* you? I sometimes ask myself when I look in the mirror. I see my body but need to remember that another, equally important part of my self-identity goes beyond physical ability or appearance.

Part of what I hope will come from this book—or my cancer experience—is others really, truly understanding that cancer, like life, is what one makes it. Some people who get cancer have a rougher physical time than others. Some people are more naturally upbeat, whether they have cancer or not. Whatever is the real experience for each person with cancer should be respected for what it is. What people with cancer should not have to worry about is how their experience is being evaluated by others.

I applaud Leahy for accurately summarizing my experience with my changing self-perceptions and others' expectations of my identity and journey because of cancer: "The cancer patient may have both the old authentic voice and an emergent voice that is also authentic…. Cancer often requires both the patient and those around her—family, caregivers, friends, colleagues—to hold in their minds two contradictory thoughts: anger and gratitude, grief and hope, and dying and living" (73). If I accept that who I was pre-cancer was valid and authentic (as well as, from my biased perspective, a host of other positive descriptors), then my post-cancer-diagnosis identity also is valid and authentic. My post-cancer self can embody oppositions and be a paradox. My emotions and responses to stimuli may change daily, and I realize that I might not always show as much gratitude or be able to explore and enjoy as many moments as I do now. However, I will still be me.

Like Townshend's introspection leading to Daltrey's memorable interpretation of "Who Are You" I would not be who I am today, for better or worse, if I had not had cancer. Without cancer, I may not have arrived at my current philosophical acceptance of the progression of life to death. I wouldn't have pragmatically put my financial affairs in order or filled my bucket list with memorable new experiences. I wouldn't count my accomplishments instead of sheep when I have insomnia. Of course, I also wouldn't look in the mirror at my sagging cheeks and puppet mouth and wonder if they are the result of normal or disease-exacerbated signs of aging. I wouldn't check whether tickets can be refunded by second parties when I plan to attend a concert or play months into the future, but then, I probably wouldn't have gone to as many plays or concerts if I expected to live another decade or had never confronted my mortality. I might not have, for example, bought a ticket to The Who's Moving On! concert and planned a weekend in Tampa in late September (during the height of hurricane season to boot) to coincide with this concert scheduled more than a year after I was expected to die. Without my diagnosis, I might not have understood that what likely is The Who's farewell tour is likely also part of my own, should I live so long. Unlike Daltrey or Townshend in their respective memoirs, I might never have attempted to put my life in perspective and reconcile who I was, publicly and privately, with who I now am if it were not for my disease. Like the lyrics and performance of "Who Are You," I have come to a point where I really want to know who I am and the significance I confer to those around me. A clearer understanding of my physical identity, past and present, helps me deal with my and everyone else's expectations about life and death with cancer.

CHAPTER 8

Abnormal
as the New Normal

When I Am Old,
I Will Be "Purple"

Writing that, as an "old" woman (I insist on the quotation marks because I keep reading that 60 is the new 40), I will definitely be purple might be prophetically dire. Turning purple/blue from lack of oxygen is not something to look forward to if my lung tumors lead to my inability to breathe. However, I otherwise embrace my definition of "being purple" that provides me with a new psychological and emotional identity reflecting my current reality. For me, being abnormal is the new normal, and my preferences, attitudes, hopes, and memories make me who I am as much as, or perhaps even more than, my physicality. I can rationalize my affinity with purple by recognizing its cultural significance in so many different ways.

In Reiki, the crown chakra at the top of the head is purple, and purple light is often envisioned for enlightenment during meditation. (When I lived in Bowling Green, Ohio, during the 1990s, I studied Reiki at a now-defunct psychic center in Toledo and, through a series of weekend workshops, became a Reiki master. Today I primarily use only a few symbols for self-healing and meditation.)

Purple has more widely socially-acceptable connotations, as well. It traditionally has been a color worn by royalty. Although I have no royal blood, this association may still be appropriate for me, given that family members have reminded me over the years that I often act like a queen and expect to be treated as visiting royalty. Once I was told that I act not like family but as a guest, expecting to be served and waited upon; likely this was a more descriptive way of telling me I am a royal pain in the arse.

In art, as a blend of red and blue, purple balances the stimulation of red with the calmness of blue; purple thus provides an appropriate color harmony that reminds me of the balance I strive to achieve between my frantic need to live fully or spontaneously and my calm awareness and appreciation of how much time I may have left. Wearing purple may make me feel not only calm but creative, spiritual, and uplifted (K. Smith).

More randomly, I shared the birthday (February 27) of violet-eyed actor Elizabeth Taylor, who favored the color purple. Our February birthstone is amethyst and birth flower is the violet. Perhaps, given all these associations and preferences, I was destined to be "purple" as a senior woman.

Being purple provides the benefit of embracing my "otherness" as part of my self-identity, because the ways that my family, friends, or "outsiders" use to define my identity may not exactly include "otherness" as a desirable quality. I may be considered "other" because of the roles I have chosen; I may be stereotyped by my job title of professor. Certainly, I have always been "other" in my family because of my less conventional choices compared with the normal achievements of my cousins or sibling. For example, I have never married or given birth to or reared a child. My career pursuits have differed from theirs: I earned a Ph.D. and became employed by more than one university, and I have traveled internationally (without making a commitment to the Navy, Army, Air Force, or Marines). My personal interests also are well outside the realm of normal pastimes of most family members, but I participate in a variety of fandoms (e.g., *Star Trek*, *Quantum Leap*, *LOST*, *Doctor Who*, *Torchwood*, *Lord of the Rings*, *Sherlock*). My initial cancer diagnosis and then my terminal illness further altered my self-identity, as well as the way that others categorize me by the choices I make regarding my treatment or the way I spend my remaining months. In my career, I am challenged by others' preconceptions of who a university teacher should be: what she should think, how she should present herself to students and colleagues, how she chooses to spend her time on campus, and whether she measures up to standards of collegiality, professionalism, and ability to guide students.

A typical example illustrates the dissonance between looking normal and really being abnormal as a teacher. In my mind, I am professional and efficient. I exude confidence and control. Yet, my body often does not cooperate with this mental self-identity or my colleagues' or students' expectations of what a professor should be. When I rush from my speech class to run to the restroom at the far end of a long hallway, my students are uncertain what to do or think. Was the speech in progress so bad that the professor bolted? What made Dr. Porter leave without explanation? Will she be back? Most important, should we wait or escape to Starbucks? Meanwhile, I struggle in the restroom and try to decide if I can make it back to class any time soon. I, too, have lots of questions: What will my students think? Did the speaker I distracted as I ran past finish the speech? How awful will this incident look on camera—and will it go viral after it's automatically posted to our course site? Was I unprofessional for running out? How much should I tell my students about my illness? Will I be able to go back to class? Can I even be a professor any longer? If I express my frustration, anger, or depression at having to leave the classroom, is that "normal" and acceptable for a cancer patient, whereas it would be deemed unprofessional for a normal teacher to show such negative emotions in front of students or colleagues? If I leave campus earlier than scheduled because I'm having a tough day physically or emotionally as a "dead" woman, is that acceptable, whereas a normal person skiving off at least once a week might receive a warning? I'm unsure how much emotion is acceptable to show on the job or whether my physical "weakness" also seems to reflect psychological or emotional weakness.

My "new normal" means that my students and I must deal with my ongoing health problems, but these types of questions about my self-identity and my performance of a work role simply do not occur in a "normal" educational setting. Therefore, after the first of what may be many such instances of my running out of the classroom, I developed a procedure to establish a "new normal" for our course: Early in the semester, I explain to my students that I have health issues that sometimes force me to leave the classroom unexpectedly. I ask them to wait 10 minutes and, if a speech is in progress, to finish. I apologize for the inconvenience and distraction but try not to feel guilty. Having cancer is not my fault. Having to bolt from a classroom is not ideal but is not my fault. After all, I carefully plan every morsel I eat or drop I drink to avoid problems during a day on campus, and the results of my preparations are inconsistent. Although I have long suspected that I would be "purple" in old age, being purple as a "dead" woman can be empowering, even in embarrassing or compromising situations, as long as I do not succumb to guilt or shame (even when I have to change clothes in a restroom). Being purple is a mindset that allows me to accept myself as I now am and to prepare myself for the me I will become before death. This shift in self-awareness and -acceptance has been a long time coming—but I suspect I would have gone purple even without a cancer diagnosis. The only difference is that I would not feel the need to explain my situation to my students.

Whereas teaching may be more a daily challenge, I can, at least theoretically, write anywhere and at any time, even around trips to the bathroom. My identity as a writer is not often challenged, in part because writing often takes place in isolation. Writers are often expected to be solitary and contemplative, or even quirky—that's part of their expected persona. Although I am not "other" by choosing to spend hours at a time writing articles or books, I differ in writing theme and style from the fiction writers in my family: Bart, Janet, and her father, mystery novelist Edward Mathis. I am more like the long-dead Day relatives my mother described as possible sources of my "writing gene." According to Mom, the Days often filled tables, chairs, and occasionally floor space with old newspapers, almanacs, and handwritten notes. She recalled a childhood visit to her mother's cousins' house and playing hide and seek around the stacks of paper. "When they needed money, they looked up some facts in an almanac and wrote another article about farming," Mom explained. "They never farmed a day in their lives, but they wrote about it." She shook her head in wonder, whether at their talent or audacity I'm not sure. Perhaps my becoming a technical writer or Bart being a journalist was due, in part, to the Days' genes filtering down a few generations, just as Mom's inability to understand why anyone would pay to read what I wrote was a likely throwback to her and her mother's interpretation of the Days' research-and-writing methods. My tendency to organize-by-stack on the dining room table must have haunted Mom, who weekly sorted receipts into neatly labeled folders filed in desk drawers.

Being "purple" post-diagnosis means I no longer feel guilty about these traits. I accept that I'm merely being "purple" when I start writing in the early afternoon and only come back to the real world when I suddenly notice it's dark. I no longer compare my writing process to that of my relatives. What people have come to expect of me as a writer—my preferences and choices about when, where, and how to express myself in prose—have not been affected by cancer yet. Writing is the one physical task that I can still accomplish relatively easily, and it reflects my psychological/emotional identity more than my physical ability to type, for example. Even when my body fails me and I may not have the energy or muscular coordination to spend hours with my laptop, I may still be able to use voice-recognition programs to translate my words into printed prose. My emotional connection to the act of writing may persist and be the most consistent aspect of my self-identity throughout my dying days. I simply may need to find more "purple" or "other" ways to accomplish the physical task of massaging words on a screen.

When I coaxed Jen into accompanying me on a weekend research trip to the North Carolina Museum of Art in Raleigh, North Carolina, in November 2018, I was fully aware that I might not live to write a book chapter about Georgia O'Keeffe, much less see it published. Nevertheless, I savored a morning viewing the special exhibition of O'Keeffe's art, as well as exulted in a relaxing Saturday afternoon that was poised between the languor of autumn and the rush of the holiday season. Jen's uncle, Gerry Crotty, became our genial weekend guide. He treated us to excellent dinners and led us through intriguing local shops, but, just as important, he visited with Jen, and they both allowed me to be myself and not worry about what others thought of the intensity of my interest in art or nature. After visiting the museum, I gushed over an old film in which O'Keeffe discusses painting near her New Mexico homestead. I watched it six times, poring over images, jotting notes, or photographing O'Keeffe quotations. Just as time consuming, outside the museum I snapped dozens of digital photos of the trees stubbornly holding on to red leaves in late November. On the flight home, Jen didn't quibble as I arranged *Southwest* magazine on my lap to click a close-up of an article useful to my ongoing research, even while passengers maneuvered around my weirdly bent elbows as I framed the shot. To Jen (and probably now to her Uncle Gerry), my obsession with research and writing is "normal" for me, and my being a more typical tourist could be cause for alarm. They accept me as just being "purple."

Like the previous chapter's question "Who are you?," which helps me come to terms with my physical identity as a body, cancer has made me question the way my "body" identity has an impact on my psychological/emotional self-identity. If I can't teach classes at ERAU, am I still a teacher? If I manage to write a book on schedule while I take chemo, does that make me more of a person—or a more successful writer—than if I met my deadline without medical distractions? Should I be prouder of that achievement than of any of the books I have written without being under the influence of chemo? If I can no longer conduct research, write, speak publicly, or serve as a faculty member, what will my identity be? (*Cancer fighter* is not the action-focused identity I seek or will ever acknowledge.)

Thus, my pragmatic self-identity has become *purple*. This classification envelops the actions of "being" purple, the beauty or attractiveness of the color purple, and the desirability to confront my and others' expectations of what it means to be a senior woman with terminal cancer. The seeds of this self-identity were planted during my childhood interactions with my paternal grandmother, but they took root more firmly in my late 40s.

In the spring of 2004, my then-department chair, Nancy Parker, and I visited Primarily Purple, an everything-purple shop in San Antonio. It was close to the Riverwalk hotel where we were attending the Popular Culture Association/Southwest Popular and American Culture Association conference, and, during a break between sessions, we window shopped. At the time, I wasn't a fanatic for the color, but purple was Nancy's favorite, and I was fascinated by the store. Of course, the shop featured t-shirts emblazoned with the first line of Jenny Joseph's famous poem, "Warning," about old ladies wearing purple. I calmly accepted the fact that, on a far-away someday when I would be old (although my students already considered me ancient at 47), I likely would wear purple—and wear it well. I had not yet begun to gain post-menopausal weight and girth, and I had never been ill beyond an occasional cold or sinus infection. Since January 2018, Joseph's approach to old age has found new life in me, and several more lines of her poem resonate as I become increasingly "purple."

In the poem, Joseph writes about youth being a sober time, and my youth and young adulthood were, with one memorable lapse, decidedly sober. I never wanted to shame my family with my behavior, and my few "wild" nights—like thoroughly enjoying the open bar at the Christmas party held by the bank where I was employed as a teller—resulted in deep familial disapproval. After I had dutifully played a selection of festive songs on the piano early in the party, I relaxed in relief—no missed notes or faltering phrasing! Sitting without a plus-one at a rear table, I decided to take up a co-worker's invitation to try a gin and tonic—more than once. When Mom and Bart picked me up after the party, my brother was tasked with directing me from the lobby to our car's remote parking spot. I think I had downed four drinks, an appalling number even for a Friday night before a weekend off work. "You smell like a distillery," Bart hissed as he pulled me toward the car. "Don't say a word on the way home." I remained silent but, given the frowns and stares during the ride and through the following morning (after my introduction to bed spins), my inebriation was loudly broadcast. As both the manager of an insurance agency across the street from my employer and a prominent bank client, at the next Rotary meeting Dad had to face the branch manager who must have seen me drunk. As a member of the downtown United Methodist Church, I had mightily sinned. As a role model for my three-years-younger brother, I had failed. As a daughter still living at home and partaking of my family's generosity, I had shamed not only myself but everyone in the household. (Only Andre, our ancient poodle, cuddled up to me that weekend. He often hung around me after he smelled spaghetti on my breath because he knew I would tie back his ears so he could enjoy the dinner leftovers as an illicit treat. Thus, he likely anticipated an exciting new taste sensation after getting a whiff of gin and tonic.) After that experience, I remained resolutely sober for several years. I lived quietly at home and worked, in succession during the next four years, as a bank teller, a deejay at a couple of adult contemporary radio stations, and a tutor at a nearby university's communication center. Only when I was 25 did I venture away from home again and enter the heady world of graduate school, professional writing, freelance consulting, and networking at business and academic conferences—where I imbibed the occasional closely monitored glass of white wine.

Like Joseph's poem suggests, however, I feel compelled not exactly to abandon sobriety—literally or figuratively—but to live a bit more spontaneously and daringly as I attain greater age. I will never be a daredevil, but I am comfortable being increasingly "purple" in my life choices of where I want to go and what I want to do—or not do—there. For example, if I decide during a research trip to Albuquerque to stay a day longer and drive to the Grand Canyon "just because," I do it. I may bemoan the lack of rest parks on I-40 between the Painted Desert National Monument exit near Winslow and Flagstaff and have to improvise a pit stop. I may exhaustedly flop into bed at 5 p.m. after a nine-hour drive (not including a one-hour time change) from Albuquerque, New Mexico, to Grand Canyon Village, Arizona. However, I also can relive a favorite childhood vacation memory when Bart and I shared the family station wagon's backseat on the journey from Indiana to California.

Like my family had done more than a half-century earlier, I stopped to marvel at the Painted Desert, Petrified Forest, and Grand Canyon. I enjoyed the cool September evenings that painted the trees just as brightly as the Painted Desert. From the gift shop, I carefully chose a piece of petrified wood to take home, as much a souvenir for Dad, Mom, and Bart, who could be with me only in spirit, as for myself. In Arizona, I entered the Grand Canyon National Park before dawn and stood with dozens of other tourists at Mather's Point, gaping at the sun's rays rising above the red rocks to gradually lighten the gaping slash in the earth before us. Driving alone across the desert was difficult, especially because I knew I would likely (and then did) face physical discomfort or problems while hiking or driving. Being purple is a recognition of the possible risks but still choosing to embrace the likely benefits of taking a once-in-a-remaining-lifetime side trip. I became drunk on independence and the beauty of nature along every mile of that trip, only sobering up when I flew home and had to return to teaching a few hours after my flight. Spontaneity is becoming a frequent travel companion, whether on a cross-country jaunt or an on-the-spot decision to head to the beach instead of going home to grade papers.

Moderation, however, must be key, even in expressions of joy at simply being alive. My excessive good humor can seem a bit over the top to others and, if I'm honest, even annoying to normal people—those who rush to get children to school on time, clean up after a pet's mess, get stuck in traffic while running late to a doctor appointment, et cetera. Whereas Pollyanna was great for Disney and Hayley Mills, the actor who received a special Oscar for playing the uber-optimistic girl on film in the early 1960s, being a Pollyanna at inopportune times can be a bit annoying. Just as Mom and Bart had disapproved of my physical intoxication following that long-ago Christmas party, Christmas season 2018 also saw me irritatingly drunk—this time on life.

On the way to a holiday chorus concert in which Thomas, Jen's nine-year-old son, would be singing that December evening, I became fascinated with the neighbors' outdoor Christmas decorations. I already felt rather giddy after having an upbeat end to the semester's classes a few hours earlier. "This is like a progressive Christmas," I chirped from the backseat. "I get to go to the concert tonight, and again on Saturday, and then there's the Sanford parade Saturday night. This week is just one big celebration!" "You're holly and jolly," Jen responded as she maneuvered through traffic. If a voice could raise a skeptical eyebrow and look askance, hers did. Whereas I had cruised to her house after a leisurely afternoon of grading final papers at a nearby Panera, she had slaved over administrative duties at the university (an especially hectic place at the end of a semester), driven her hour-long I-4 commute home, fed everyone dinner, kept apart new puppy Bailey and growly older (and long-established pet) Bowie, wrangled children into band or chorus uniforms, herded the carload of people going to the concert into the car, and now had to find a parking place and get everyone inside and seated within the next few minutes. It was a typical Mom evening—but I, who have never been a Mom, typical or purple, only needed to pay attention to the blow-up Santas and reindeer out my window. I wasn't offended by Jen's response, just aware of my super-happy tone, and chuckled, "That was kind of obnoxious, wasn't it?" "I didn't say that," Jen calmly replied—but we both knew it kind of was. At times my overjoyed oversharing resembles actor Christopher Plummer's description of working on *The Sound of Music* (1965): "It's like getting hit over the head every day with a Hallmark Card" (Cosgrave).

Sometimes my "new normal" purple personality is a little too perky, not from trying to convince myself that all is well, but because I am aware of the joy of seeing holiday lights and attending a school concert when I have no claim as a parent or grandparent to be there. I likely over-respond because I don't have such biological ties and feel especially grateful to be included. Heather lived far away from me during much of her youth, and, because of the distance between Florida and Ohio, I now miss her children's school and holiday events. I love Heather (and Levi and Ava), but I'm not actively involved in their daily lives. For better or worse for the Wojtons, Jen and Chris have allowed me to become an "auntie" to their children, and Joy and Carlos similarly have made sure that Nico and Roman include Auntie Nette among the many biological and by-marriage aunts and uncles. Without this extended family, I would never have the opportunity to go to Thursday night holiday concerts or Saturday evening parades, to sing "Happy Birthday" at parties throughout the year, to jump into a backyard pool or hot tub during a summer afternoon visit to Joy's, or to join the kids on ride after ride at the Magic Kingdom. For all those opportunities to become part of a family (and, in true "auntie" fashion, leave when the kids argue or get cranky), I am immensely thankful—but I sometimes should tone it down just a wee bit.

Joseph's poem also warns that a purple old lady is allowed to get fatter, and so I have. Remaining vegetarian, even after 15 years of habit, became too difficult when hospital staff admonished me that I needed more protein following surgeries. My body also gleefully rejected most vegetables and fruits as too difficult to digest following my ileostomy reversal. Instead, for months, it preferred white-meat chicken slices and white bread—or else I did penance in the bathroom for hours for the sin of sneaking bites of strawberries or salad. A rather gross scene from *The Favourite* (2018) humbles me because I can relate to early 18th-century English queen Anne (Olivia Colman) stuffing her face with blue cake, only (as she had been previously warned would happen) for it to make her immediately and violently ill. She vomits into a bucket provided by a helpful servant, then viciously takes another bite of cake. Sometimes I just want what I want in the moment, even if I know that I am likely to be unable to leave the house for the rest of the day.

As a result of my "purple" attitude toward food and drink, my closet now contains jeans in three sizes so that I have something to wear, no matter my current level of indulgence. When I need to justify my urge for chocolate-covered almonds or chicken taquitos, I remind myself that a lifestyle of never touching nicotine, limiting sugar and carbs, and avoiding meat did not render me cancer free (or even a size 8 or less). Sipping champagne while I watch *Doctor Who* or munching M&Ms instead of having a salad for dinner probably is not increasing my lifespan and only adding to my waist-span, but I am more inclined to "go purple" if, in the moment, my culinary indulgence is soulfully enriching.

Perhaps the universe even encouraged my going purple at this time in my life. Each year, the Pantone company (best known for its patented Color Matching System, most notably used in the printing industry) selects its color of the year. Appropriately for me, the color of the year in 2018, the year of my terminal diagnosis, was ultra violet. In many ways, purple—in a variety of shades, not just Pantone's #18–3838— became my trademark in 2018 and brought together many elements of my past and present.

I suppose I shouldn't be surprised that I gravitated toward purple when I passed 60. As much as I fought against my genetic inheritance and its implication that I would be most like the person I most closely resemble, I have ended up very much like my paternal grandmother, Mary Pauline Staples Porter, more popularly known as Polly. From her I received the shape of my face—narrower forehead, prominent cheekbones, and the hint of a widow's peak. She passed along those attributes to my father, who gave them to me, along with his light blue Porter eyes— a stark contrast from Polly's deep brown. Like Dad and Mom-Ma Polly, I earned more pride than money from my career and learned to establish schedules for formal familial visits. Especially when I was younger, say, 25 to 50, I privileged work to family. I enjoyed spending my "free" time on a work-related project: writing a book, editing journals, creating technical communication workshops, and going to as many academic conferences as possible in as many locales as a university's (and my) budget could take me. I seldom let anyone invade my home (mostly because I am a terrible housekeeper and feel uncomfortable revealing my ancient, dust-covered furnishings and stacks of notes to anyone, including blood kin). Mom-Ma Polly—the first person I ever knew who hired someone to clean her house once a week while she was at work—invited her only son, his wife, and two children for either Thanksgiving or Christmas dinner each year. My parents discussed which holiday would be spent in the little shotgun-style house on Indiana Street, and Mom-Ma Polly planned accordingly.

My grandparents lived modestly and had worked hard to join the middle class. They lived in the home where my father was born in 1933 and worked 40 hours a week, most years without any vacation time. Pop-Pa became employed at an electric company after leaving his job at the brewery when he joined the Baptist church; he also became a proud union representative. Mom-Ma Polly was a receptionist/clerk in an optometrist's office. Until I was five or six, the Christmas goose or Thanksgiving duck most likely had been shot by either Dad or Pop-Pa, who hid in a blind on a lake or river in southern Indiana until the unlucky bird answered a fake call. More than once Mom double-checked the holiday meat before Bart or I tucked into the feast, making sure no pieces of buckshot had slipped past Mom-Ma Polly's scrutiny. Despite serving the free bird, Mom-Ma Polly liked to make these once-a-year gatherings special with store-bought extras. Every place setting was adorned with a nut cup filled with cashews and pecans. Dessert included either a holly-sprigged, coconut-covered ice cream ball (aka "snowball") or a mint-flavored ice cream shaped like Santa Claus or a Christmas tree. After dinner, Bart and I retired to Dad's former bedroom, now the TV room, to watch *Wonderful World of Disney* or *A Charlie Brown Christmas* while the grownups talked until it was time to go home around 8.

Despite all this formality and structure, Mom-Ma Polly had a carefully managed "wild" side that showed up in innovative ways. Since the days when my father worked by day and attended classes by night to attain a business degree at Evansville College (later University of Evansville), Mom-Ma Polly loved going to the school's Purple Aces basketball games. By the mid–1960s, she and my grandfather achieved the status of season ticket holders. Mom-Ma Polly faithfully donned her favorite purple sweater or skirt and white go-go boots to attend games at Evansville's Stadium. (She bought me a pair of matching boots, which was sublime gear for an eight-year-old.) She also decided to paint the bathroom in her favorite shade of purple: lavender. Not only was the tiny room repainted, but she appliqued pink flamingos at the back of the sink. For all her conservative Baptist beliefs, she found ways to uniquely express her individuality.

Shortly after I graduated from high school, Mom-Ma Polly was diagnosed with lung cancer, which was especially shocking because she had never touched a cigarette. The Staples family lived on a farm in northwestern Kentucky in the early 1900s, where Polly, the second of five children, was born in 1907. My grandmother never wanted to talk about the dead; hence, I have no information beyond Ancestry.com hints regarding Dad's ancestors. I don't know if anyone else died from cancer or even if that diagnosis could have been made back then. Mom-Ma Polly was briefly in the hospital in autumn 1975, just as I began my first year at the local university, but I don't remember that she took any kind of treatment or special medication. No one ever told me that she wouldn't recover or was expected to survive less than a year, although, at 18, I probably should have realized that lung cancer was a death sentence. Although I obliviously thrived in my exciting new world of living alone and unsupervised, I occasionally visited my grandparents only a few miles away. As I sat at the kitchen table sipping a soda, I saw nothing out of the ordinary beyond my grandparents no longer going to work and having time to chat in the middle of the afternoon. By then, Mom-Ma Polly was in her late 60s, so seeing her "retired" was not that unexpected. Taking her ticket to accompany Pop-Pa to Aces games was. Even then, I expected Mom-Ma to continue living—dying of cancer was not yet in my understanding of the possible, much less the probable.

As my grandmother's health gradually deteriorated, she spent more days on the porch. She no longer wore purple; her pajamas were as pale as her skin. The last time I visited her she sat bundled in blankets in early May. The weather was warm enough for her beloved roses to bloom, but she no longer could venture into the garden to sniff their heady fragrance. During that final visit, her left foot slid off a footstool, and she didn't have the strength to lift it. Mom tearfully returned the wayward limb to its resting place. A month later, two days shy of her 69th birthday, Mom-Ma Polly died quietly of cancer—just as Dad would do 17 years later, and Bart 22 years after that. These days I often wonder when I will follow the family tradition.

For all that I can now see my physical resemblance to my grandmother and have long followed in her workaholic steps, only recently— when purple became my new favorite color—did I admit we had anything in common. After all, she and I never were close, and I was far from her favorite, a fun fact that Bart and I discussed during some of our final visits, as we analyzed our common childhood experiences.

Mom-Ma Polly preferred boys, and she doted on Dad, her only son, and Bart, her only grandson. She was a good "country" cook who enjoyed baking and plied the men in her life with deliciously lard-laden peach cobblers or angel food cakes slathered with real whipped cream and dusted with bits of Heath bars. Although, unlike Bart, I didn't sit in the kitchen talking with her or watching her cook, I enjoyed the infrequent opportunity to sit on the backyard swing, breaking green beans that Mom-Ma Polly later turned into wonderfully baconed bites of heaven. However, whereas Pop-Pa, Dad, and Bart could stay slim, year after year, while savoring this richness, I had inherited Mom's metabolism and increasingly round midsection. I didn't meet the requirements for being the good granddaughter Mom-Ma Polly envisioned: a pretty young woman with an hour-glass figure inherited from the Staples women, as well as an excellent "from scratch" cook and homemaker who fit into the modern world by having an office job. She appreciated my parents' expectation that I would get a college degree, following along the path paved by my first-generation-college-student father. However, being a "catch" was also important. Although Mom-Ma Polly might have enjoyed the "purple" tendencies that separated her from many women of her generation, such as a managerial office job and her own money, deep down she was still a traditional farm girl who lived the truth of the saying, "The best way to a man's heart is through his stomach." Thus, at 12, I tried to get excited about the trendy clothes Mom-Ma Polly wanted to buy me when she took me on our only back-to-school shopping trip. Both of us were unhappy when I couldn't fit into anything in the teen shops. Stunned by my first migraine and quickly returned home hours ahead of schedule from that fateful shopping trip, I only succeeded in feeling too different from the woman who wanted to spoil me and show me off. Mom-Ma Polly, who never mothered a daughter, had no idea what to do with her granddaughter, especially a rotund mass of preteen insecurity who didn't fit the master plan. Perhaps if I had been more assertively "purple" back then, she might have been able to relate to the "otherness" in me. After all, as a young woman, she determinedly moved off the farm and to the city to find work (even if she also wanted a husband), and she derived a large part of her identity from her career outside the home and her basketball fandom, which were not common identity markers for a woman in her 50s or 60s in southern Indiana in the early 1970s. I sometimes wonder if Mom-Ma Polly would feel relieved if she knew that I eventually followed in her purple footsteps to become a career woman who looks strikingly like her (albeit one who couldn't bake a peach cobbler to save her life).

My grandmother and I ironically ended up with more similarities than I ever could have imagined, such as eccentric tastes on which to splurge discretionary income or the mutual experience of retirement because of a terminal cancer diagnosis. Whereas Mom-Ma Polly painted the bathroom purple and donned her beloved basketball team's colors for each winter home game, my purple passion has taken a different form. I, too, like wearing purple, but I prefer theme-park t-shirts and Vejas' lilac-colored vegan sneakers. However, we both discovered the joys of hair color.

Until Mom-Ma Polly could no longer leave home, she faithfully visited a salon to maintain her short blonde hairstyle. She may have wanted to believe that blondes have more fun when, in the early 1960s, she banished her brown locks for good and decided never, ever to go grey. That also became my mantra, despite some predicted complications. Before I began radiation treatments in summer 2016, a counselor at the cancer center explained that I would lose my hair but—good news!—my insurance would pay for two wigs a year. She proceeded to show me a variety of colors and styles to help me get my head around the fact that I would lose my hair and require scalp glue. Instead of scheduling a wig-fitting session, I made an appointment with Danielle, a member of my supportive extended Carney-Wojton-Arias family, and a genius of coloring and styling. I realized that my shoulder-length bob would go—one way or another. Proactively, I asked that my hair be reduced to head-hugging pixie length. Contrary to the counselor's prediction, I never lost my hair (just my dignity, part of my colon, my appendix, and my left ovary) because of cancer treatments or surgeries. A few weeks before my 60th birthday, I embraced the Cold War anti–McCarthy slogan "Better red than dead" (the flip side of McCarthyism's "Better dead than red") and traded blonde for bright copper. Fresh from a terminal diagnosis a year later, I went purple, and, during the following months, Danielle and I experimented with highlights ranging from lavender to magenta to violet, the shade I ultimately preferred.

On one of my bucket-list trips, other women on our Scandinavian cruise approached me to tell me how my purple hair shone in the sunlight or even (a favorite compliment) looked "whimsical." Female tour guides confided that they wished they could wear an "unnatural" hair color on the job—and, indeed, I am pleased that my employment has no such stipulation. My hair also invited questions that were humorous to me but apparently serious to the asker. One woman riding the same tour bus as I twice in one week noticed that my hair was color-coordinated with my cardigan or blouse each time she saw me; she asked whether I color my hair each evening to match my clothes the next day. (The answer, by the way, is no.) Back home in Ormond Beach, servers have come over to whisper that they love my hair color or tell me that I am brave for dyeing my hair purple. Colleagues stop by my office to check out my latest shade and encourage me to embrace my stylistic creativity. I seem far more interesting and garner much more public attention now that I am purple.

Being purple is reflected in more than my changes in hair color or clothing. My "purple" attitude empowers me. I would rather be called brave for changing my hair color than for living with cancer; I can choose my hair color, but I have no choice of diagnosis. Taking control of even one tiny aspect of my life—such as how to style my hair—makes a huge difference in my ability to live happily day to day. I take pride in my choices and can better accept the aspects of life over which I am slowly losing control. Sometime soon I will not be able to manage my hair color-day ritual: drive an hour to the Thornton Park area of Orlando; enjoy the sunshine and a latte at the little French bakery down the street from the salon; collaborate with Danielle on the ever-important decisions regarding color and cut; and spend before- or after-salon time with Jen. However, I *can* do that now—and I can optimistically make an appointment to follow this familiar routine in six weeks. Living "purple" is life itself—quirky, optimistic, age defying, death defying. Now that I am an old(er) woman, I do more than wear purple. I thank poets like Jenny Joseph and women of another generation, like Polly Porter, for inspiring me to *be* purple.

CHAPTER 9

Great (or Not-So-Great) Expectations—Mine and Everyone Else's

Like young Philip Pirrip, better known as Pip, in Charles Dickens' *Great Expectations* (1861), I received shocking news and developed great expectations about what my future should be as a result of my altered fortunes. Several years into his apprenticeship as a blacksmith, Pip received official word that his financial fortunes would improve: he had come into money from an unnamed benefactor and immediately left his employment to set upon a great adventure befitting his new life as a gentleman. However, among Dickens' hundreds of following pages, Pip learns that his new status does not mesh with his great expectations—or the great expectations others (such as his benefactor and family) have for him when he first receives word that his circumstances have changed. Yet, by the end of his story, Pip has achieved a measure of peace after great suffering. Life may not have been what he or anyone else expected, but he eventually learns to live on his own terms.

I can certainly relate to Pip. My shocking news was not wealth but cancer, with its expectations for treatments, surgeries, success rates, and percentages of likely survival by year. These shifting fortunes shifted further a couple of years later because of a diagnosis of metastatic tumors and a prognosis of six months to p-o-s-s-i-b-l-y a year of remaining life, with lots of gruesome events along the journey leading to death. As a result of this official word, my fortunes definitely changed; after all, the retirement money I had saved (not counting the Social Security account I likely would never be able to touch) would provide for me nicely for six months, even a year or two if I could count on insurance to pay my medical expenses. (My cashed reserves would not come close to supporting me for the expected 20 years after "normal" retirement in one's mid–60s, but now running out of money was no longer a concern. Huzzah!) Even better than money, my benefactor friends at work gave me time away from my duties so that I could set upon a great adventure befitting my new life (first stop, Reykjavik). However, during my time as one of the walking dead, I, like Pip, discovered that this new life does not mesh with my or others' great (or not-so-great) expectations. My story has not yet ended, but I expect—perhaps, hopefully, to be wrong about these expectations, too—that I, like Pip, have more suffering ahead before my final peace, The End.

The expectations I have encountered as someone with cancer have had a powerful impact on me. Although I can read death statistics and refer to cost estimates to gain some knowledge of what to expect when I am expecting to die, especially in the final weeks or days before my final breath, the most enlightening (and sometimes haunting or horrifying) information is based on the way family members died and the comments made by everyone from family members or friends to healthcare professionals to random people whose lives intersect with mine.

Four "horrors" from my observations of familial cancer patients have, unfortunately, formed the basis of my expectations for the very end of life:

1. My paternal grandmother's death

In 1979, Mom-Ma Polly lost her battle with lung cancer midway through the year. By then, she couldn't move without help. If she didn't move at all, she had less pain. When her imminent death became obvious to Pop-Pa, he called an ambulance to take her to the hospital, where nothing could be done. Pop-Pa called Dad in Ohio to let him know what was happening, but there was not enough time to drive the eight hours to Evansville to say goodbye, and direct flights between Lima, Ohio, and Evansville, Indiana, didn't exist. Mom-Ma Polly died alone in an isolated hospital room. When I saw her during the funeral viewing two days later, she looked as shrunken as a dried-apple doll, her blonde wig perched precariously on her head. I was pleased that Pop-Pa thought to have her dressed in a pantsuit—I had never seen her wear a dress and wanted her to retain some individuality in defiance of the homogenizing treatment she had received as a cancer patient. I don't want to die alone in a hospital room—yet that is one typical expectation about a cancer patient's end of life.

2. My maternal grandmother's death

Mom-Ma Margie, Dad, and Bart spent their last days at home. In June 1987, Mom-Ma Margie rather suddenly (it seemed to me) became hospitalized. Mom and I drove from Ohio to Indiana to visit her, but Mom-Ma didn't recognize us. Her demeanor was especially troubling for me; I thought I was her favorite granddaughter. Mom-Ma slyly tried to win my favor by telling me she liked my summer dress and then asking if I would help her escape. I had no idea (and have never been able to figure out) why she no longer seemed mentally capable of taking care of herself. Up to that time, she had lived alone. She hadn't fallen or visibly been sick—or at least no one sent the news to Ohio. With nothing we could do to help her (I avoided the Great Escape, much to my grandmother's annoyance, and thus was no help at all), Mom and I drove back to Ohio. At the end of July, Mom was called to Evansville to help care for Mom-Ma Margie at her tiny brick house on Chestnut Street. The daughters who still lived in Indiana (Hazel, Helen, and Bettye) were already there when Mom arrived, and the death-watch experience was horrific. Not all the sisters agreed with each other on good days, so some general bickering was expected. Someone later told me my grandmother had stomach cancer, but she had never received medication or treatment. Apparently she had been sent home from the hospital to die; nothing would help her. Still, my understanding that my mother and aunts had no pain medication to give her and that my grandmother moaned for days, at times thinking she was birthing one of her six children, haunts me. On the day before her death, Mom-Ma Margie talked frequently to her first husband, her children's father, who died only six months after my mother's birth in 1932. She addressed Jim by name and answered his questions with more lucidity than she interacted with her daughters. Although Mom-Ma Margie was surrounded by four children in her bedroom as she died, her passing was not serene. The torment of her pain and dementia was matched by the stifling early August heat of both a home with only one overworked living room air conditioner and the intensity of her daughters' grief and dissent. My expectation is that dying at home is more peaceful for the one leaving, as well as the left behind. Mom-Ma Margie's passing depressingly defied that expectation.

3. My father's death

I vividly remember Dad rallying on a Friday night in mid–August 1993 before he died on Sunday: talking with visitors, eating his favorite cherry pie that Aunt Irene had baked from scratch, commenting that our dinner of chicken and rice was delicious. Dad mostly stayed in the hospital bed placed in the sitting room at the back of the house, close to the kitchen and with a view to the lake and the boat he had only driven twice around it. He liked his morphine pills, and, as the cancer quickly spread from his lungs to his spine, colon, and brain, lost all sense of time and kept asking for more pills hours before he could take the next dose. It was therefore a pleasant surprise when Dad seemed close to his pre-cancer self while eating dinner and chatting with visitors on that Friday night I had flown in from Ohio. Yet, after everyone but Mom, Aunt Bonnie (who had traveled from Dallas earlier in the week to help Mom for a few days), and I had left, Dad deteriorated once again. He hallucinated under the influence of the pain-dulling morphine, and each of us tried to reassure him. I didn't sleep during the next 24 hours because he didn't trust anyone but the few family members he recognized and worried that strangers would enter the house. Mom had her own health problems to worry about and couldn't care for my father alone.

On Saturday, when I drove Aunt Bonnie to the Orlando airport, she told me directly that my father had only a few days left, at most. I still found that verdict difficult to believe, even though his doctor's initial prognosis was three months, and Dad had lived two weeks past that point. Only two days earlier I had packed plenty of shorts and t-shirts for my Florida trip; I didn't think I would need any formal clothes to hang around the house or run errands for a few weeks. Likely I was in denial; definitely I didn't know that those at the end of life could rally just before dying. All the way back to Fruitland Park, I gravely considered Aunt Bonnie's words. I had never seen someone die—she had. Aunt Bonnie also had a habit of telling me what I needed to know, and I felt closer to her than to most other relatives. Instead of rushing back to my parents' house, I pulled into a grocery's parking lot and chose a spot at the end of a row. After I bought a couple of fruity wine coolers, I slumped in the car to chug them before I went back to confront life and death with my parents. Fortifying myself with cheap fake wine didn't seem like a viable long-term plan, as I wanted to be cognizant of everything Dad said or did, even if he was not.

On Sunday, around noon, Dad moaned, "Oh, I'm dying." He took one last dose of his morphine pills. Then he asked Mom if he could stay at home—knowing all that implied—and she agreed. Dad died a few hours later, without saying another word but presumably without pain. My preference is to die at home, pain free, but I don't know if I want loved ones around me or to spare them the ordeal of watching that last breath. I don't know if dying quietly at home is a realistic expectation for me, but, even though it's not ideal for those left behind, it's my favorite scenario among the ways that my family died.

4. My brother's death

In early July 2015, during one of our many phone conversations, I talked with Bart about the just-past July 4 holiday. He enthused that his dear friend Shaun Zuver had visited, and Bart's family (Nancy, Heather, and Levi) and Shaun's family (Lorraine and Suzi) enjoyed a holiday picnic in the backyard. The only problem was a persistent squirrel that kept dropping twigs onto the table from an overhead tree branch. Bart notoriously fought the squirrels that terrorized birds trying to lunch at the feeder outside his window. Even at night, squirrel bandits broke into the feeder to scatter songbird blend all over the grass for easier gorging. Despite the squirrel attack during the picnic, Bart was thankful that he could be carried outside to enjoy the sunshine and share the meal. A couple of days after that phone call, I texted Bart to see which flight the following week would arrive at the most convenient time for our next visit. As I had done a month earlier, I wanted to make a quick trip to Columbus to see Bart. I received a text (which, I later learned, was sent by Nancy on Bart's behalf) and printed my reservation. Later that afternoon, Nancy called. She immediately, tearfully apologized and, when I asked why, told me Bart was dead. After a morning medical appointment, Bart and Nancy returned home. (A nurse later told Nancy that, on the day Bart died, she thought he had a few more weeks, or she would have prepared her and called Heather to be at Bart's bedside.) Going outside the house was always an ordeal for Bart, as he didn't have a wheelchair (insurance wouldn't cover one), and his strength and balance were precarious on good days. Weeks earlier, he had fallen into a rose bush, breaking branches and his pride, when he lost his balance trying to walk to the front door. On the day he died, there were no such mishaps, but Bart complained of feeling weird, similar to the onslaught of a migraine. For months he managed his cancer pain without receiving morphine and taking only higher strength aspirin. On that day, he declined migraine pills and said he would nap for a little while. While Nancy worked around the house, Bart died in his sleep.

My hope is that I die peacefully at home, and I can't help but wonder if Bart decided to slip away without causing Nancy or Heather the agony of watching him take his last breath. This final peace was hard won after months of being nauseous or unable to eat, being cold most of the time, suffering weakness that kept him in his recliner in front of the television and next to the window overlooking the backyard, dealing with unrelieved pain of tumors large enough he could feel them in his liver, and seeing his 55-year-old body turn into that of a 90-year-old.

Unfortunately, Bart's end-of-life experience is my expectation of what happens during the final months or weeks of a cancer patient's life. Like Bart, I have colorectal cancer that has metastasized and therefore expect that my deterioration will be similar to his. My worst case scenario is that I will die (1) isolated in an impersonal care facility; (2) without medication to ease pain; and (3) causing fear or panic in friends or family because of the way my body expires. The rumor that there are no happy cancer stories has not yet become my reality, but I expect that something similar can or will happen to me—just because that is my family's collective experience. In the meantime, I am doing everything possible to plan an ending that, although it may not be happy, is peaceful and life affirming. So far, Bart's story is the most optimistic scenario for me.

As I've mentioned throughout this book, popular culture—especially film—helps provide the running movie in my mind when I depict cancer patients or their carers. Not only *Third Star* (2010) but three other films feed my expectations of what life will become for me or those who love me: *Terms of Endearment* (1983), *The Judge* (2014), and *Ode to Joy* (2018).

Of course, *Terms of Endearment* sets the standard for many viewers' expectations of those with a cancer diagnosis. As the film (and the cancer) progresses, Debra Winger's Emma Horton becomes little more than a body in a hospital bed. The film's emphasis on the relationship between Emma and her mother, Aurora Greenway (Shirley MacLaine), then shifts the focus to Aurora, who becomes a fierce advocate for her daughter's care and agrees to become guardian to her three grandchildren. Who can forget Aurora's strident demand for Emma to receive her overdue shot of morphine? The depiction of Emma as bedridden and in pain is one that haunts me. However, Emma rallies to tell her children goodbye and to show them that she understands and loves them—and wants them to feel no guilt about what they did or didn't say or do while she was alive. I can agree with that part of the film, although being that coherent so close to death isn't guaranteed. Anything that I need to say to others had best be said now, before my loved ones question even more the likelihood of cancer altering my ability to think logically or express what I really think or want.

Whereas Emma stars in primarily a "cancer story," cancer patients in *The Judge* and *Ode to Joy* are peripheral characters related to main characters who become carers but also have other plot-based reasons for starring in the story. In *The Judge*, the title character is hard-nosed retired small-town judge Joseph Palmer (Robert Duvall), who is estranged from his son, flashy big-city lawyer Hank (Robert Downey, Jr.). The plot revolves around Hank returning to his childhood home to clear his father of a murder charge. What interested (and sometimes scared) me, however, was the secret that the judge tries to keep from his son: he has cancer and is undergoing chemotherapy. Every couple of weeks, a friend drives Joseph to his treatment, but the treatments themselves are mysterious things, kept well off screen. (To be fair, there is no plot-driven reason why chemo would or should take up screen time in this film.) Nonetheless, its omission only fueled further questions about what takes place during these treatments and if, in real life, the judge could keep them quite so secret. Wouldn't he feel tired or look pale? Wouldn't even his estranged son notice something off about his father—or the lied-about nature of the periodic trips with his friend?

At the time I watched a weekday matinee of *The Judge*, Bart had been diagnosed with colorectal cancer and had surgery to remove a tumor but, at least to my mind then, was going to recover from cancer. In fact, I hoped to escape thinking about Bart's illness by going to a movie. Little did I know that "cancer" was a co-star; however, in hindsight, the insertion of a cancerous character should be more commonplace in films. Rather than centering the plot on disease or someone with it, films should include characters with cancer as part of increasing diversity. After all, many, many audience members know someone with cancer or have it themselves.

Back in 2014, I lacked details about what happens during chemo or how debilitating Bart's recovery had or would become. Undoubtedly, Bart didn't want to worry me, and, because I was his sister, he hesitated in providing gruesome details about his erratically healing digestive system. Thus, when I watched a scene in which the stoic, proud judge loses bowel control and tries unsuccessfully to manage a shower, I was shocked. Was this what Bart was dealing with? The humiliation of this scene, in which the son has to help his father stand and clean up in the shower, graphically illustrates this cancer patient's frustration and vulnerability—things he tries to hide from everyone. Only much later, when I replayed this scene multiple times in my life and shower (but without RDJ to soap me up), did I move from horror to acceptance, repulsion to pragmatism. Although I've tried not to broadcast the frequency or severity of my "accidents" at home, like the judge, I've learned to simply get on with the business of cleaning up myself and whatever room I soiled, hosing down my body and relying on Scrubbing Bubbles to eradicate the evidence. Like the judge, I prefer to deal with those kinds of situations myself, rather than rely on anyone's help. Having cancer can be dehumanizing, and neither the judge nor I want to be perceived as weak and needy. My reality (and the judge's) had been starkly depicted on screen, not as entertainment but as horror and, more important to the plot, a pathway by which father and son grow closer and realize that they both are flawed and vulnerable men, albeit in very different ways.

Acceptance of cancer and trying to come to grips with death-by-cancer is a continuing theme in the life of Francesca (Morena Baccarin), a woman who seems always to choose the wrong men. When she meets Charlie (Martin Freeman), she feels a genuine spark, but he is keeping a secret from her. He has cataplexy, a disease that causes him to fall asleep/lose consciousness if he allows himself to feel a strong emotion;

in his case, joy is a specific trigger. Therefore, Charlie limits his exposure to anything that might make him happy by reciting a litany of terrible images or stabbing his toe with a strategically placed thumbtack in his shoe. When Charlie dares to attempt a date with Francesca, he literally falls for her when she asks him to come up to her place—Charlie tumbles down stairs as he loses consciousness and, hours later, awakens in a hospital suffering from contusions and a concussion. Although Charlie's condition and the way he lives with a disease with no cure provide the humor and drama in this rom-com, Francesca's story is just as harrowing to someone like me. Her mother died of breast cancer, and her second-mom/aunt is undergoing chemo for the same form of cancer. When Francesca was in high school, she spent a wonderful summer in New York with her Aunt Sylvia (Jane Curtin), only to realize later that she could thank her mother's secretive months in chemotherapy for her holiday. Francesca is well aware that what has happened to her mom and is happening to her aunt may very well happen to her. She knows what to expect—and it's not pretty. Although Aunt Sylvia is one of those plucky cancer patients with a dirty sense of humor and a diligently pursued bucket list, she also needs a carer. She texts Francesca to tell her that, for example, she's vomiting a lot or that the results of her latest scans show her cancer has metastasized in her liver. Now-single Sylvia is fortunate, however; Francesca lives with her and can check on her or accompany her to chemo. (I was impressed that the hospital's chemo-room setting looked realistic, from my experience: a bare room with a line of faux leather recliners and bagged poles.) Despite their range of medical challenges, Francesca and Charlie learn how to take their current and potential illnesses in stride as they navigate their way toward happiness. The audience understands that Aunt Sylvia doesn't have long to live—her absence from the film's final scene a clear indicator that she has died.

Two reactions to cancer are my takeaway from this film. I find it remarkable that Charlie compassionately listens to Francesca's fears about losing her aunt and doesn't seem squeamish about dealing with Sylvia's prognosis. Unlike his well-meaning but often clueless brother, who tries to reassure Francesca that her aunt will be OK and runs away when Francesca tries to explain what it's like to be her aunt's carer, Charlie accepts the reality that cancer is awful for both patients and carers.

My second reaction comes from sitting through "cancer scenes" next to friends or family who know that I've taken chemo and I'm dying from cancer. Even those who talk candidly with me about my disease sometimes automatically stiffen in their seats and feel uncomfortable when cancer is unexpectedly forced into their line of sight. They are sad, and they don't know what to do or say to make things better. I can relate— I had the same involuntary reaction to everyone else's cancer when I was cancer free.

A similar typical "shock" reaction occurred a few days after receiving my terminal diagnosis, when I felt awkward watching *Three Billboards Outside Ebbing, Missouri* (2017) with my friends. Although Woody Harrelson's Sheriff Willoughby isn't the focal point of the story, he is a well-developed character—and he happens to be terminally ill with pancreatic cancer. In one scene, while talking with main character Mildred (Frances McDormand), Willoughby's cough spews blood on Mildred's face. Both horrified and embarrassed, Willoughby apologizes, but Mildred almost immediately recovers from the shock and uses the moment to heal their fractured (and fractious) relationship. No longer is she an angry woman seeking justice—and going to great, sometimes illegal lengths to pursue it. Instead, she becomes a supportive friend who helps put Willoughby at ease. In a subsequent hospital scene, Willoughby decides to leave for home as soon as possible, rather than seeking palliative care. Thus, it isn't too big a surprise that he chooses to take charge of his death before cancer can beat him to it. However, perhaps I reacted a little too enthusiastically about the way Sheriff Willoughby embraces his last day, doing everything he loves with his family, before blowing off his head. My friends and I automatically caught our breaths as he carefully prepared to die so as to leave as little mess as possible, but I perceived their thoughts weren't focused solely on the film. We sat together awkwardly, united not only through watching the film but relating its "cancer scenes" to my prognosis. I applaud Willoughby's idea of living fully and normally for as long as possible, but I felt compelled to alleviate my friends' possible concern that I might someday choose suicide.

Ode to Joy has such "cancer awareness" moments that stunned my friends, or even me (although I tried to be cool about the situation). Cancer-themed scenes are especially difficult to watch with friends because they momentarily pull us out of the characters' story to focus on the drama going on within my life. Yet, how wonderful it is for me to see a character like Charlie, who is terribly flawed and sometimes cruel because of his expectations of his disease and others' reactions to it but is pragmatic and genuine in his reaction to Francesca's and Sylvia's cancer stories.

What stands out for me in each of these films is that the cancer-stricken characters are aware of their disease and prognosis. These are not happy cancer stories where ill characters receive a reprieve or miraculously are cured. These characters suffer and die, whether on camera right in front of the audience or in an implied future beyond the scope of the film. Premature, tragic death is a common expectation, on film or in real life.

Terms of Endearment, The Judge, and *Ode to Joy* also represent different stages of my awareness of people with cancer, long before I became one. (I could stage my cancer awareness just as meticulously as my oncologist stages my cancer cells.) At one time or another, I could have been Hank, Francesca, or Charlie. Now I am closer to Emma, Joseph, and especially to irreverent, straightforward Sylvia. I see progress in ways these few films portray cancer on screen, with greater realism and grossness being shown on camera. More important, I have become more critical as well as more understanding of my and others' reactions to and expectations of people with cancer because of these films.

My expectations for my end of life may be bleak at this point in my cancer journey, but I feel more positively that I cannot or should not automatically succumb to others' expectations for me. Almost the minute Jen and I left my oncologist's office after receiving my unpleasant prognosis, I became aware of public, professional, and familial expectations regarding my present and future. The main expectations I have come to identify over time fall into several distinct categories related to my career and employment, independence, rationality, and religious or spiritual beliefs; almost every important aspect of living comes under fresh scrutiny from the time crunch presented by my prognosis.

Unlike my gloom regarding the ways my family died from cancer, I become downright feisty and irreverent when I am presented with others' expectations of what I should or should not do and how my philosophy meshes with theirs. Probably I am sometimes way too cranky about others' well-meaning concern, and I do want to hear what other people think or can advise. I'm thankful, for example, for Jen's guidance and assistance regarding my employment and career identity, Mike Perez's many voicemails and conversational reminders that so many people love and are willing to help me, Joy's and Carlos' knowledge and recommendations about legal matters, Janet's or Genie's dedication in checking on me and offering to fly to Florida to help, and Heather's and Nancy's willingness to rearrange work and childcare in order to travel on short notice (with two small children) so we can spend time together in Florida. Mostly as a way to deflect the seriousness of others' expectations and their deep hold on me, I turn to my strange and often inappropriate sense of humor to deal with the tension between what I want/think/believe and what others want for me, think about my situation, and believe is in my best interest.

Expectations for cancer patients, even Stage 4 colorectal cancer patients, can set up those with a terminal illness for surprise, disappointment, or even anger. However, others' expectations also have provided a catalyst for turning me into the Little Engine That Could, just to defy them. In the past two years, I devised a "Greatest Hits" compilation of my Top Four for Stage 4—my four favorite experiences in dealing with my and others' perceptions about or reactions to rectal cancer.

- The kind older woman (likely in her late 70s) who drove me to one radiation treatment is a volunteer with the American Cancer Society and a more-than-five-year cancer survivor. She attempted to make small talk on our way to the treatment center. "What kind of cancer do you have, dear?" she gently inquired. "Colorectal," I replied. Her curiosity got the better of her a few seconds later. "Oh. Hmm. Is your tumor more colon or more rectal?" "Rectal," I replied. Again there was a short pause. "Hmmm. I wonder how you got that?" My mind irreverently pictured myself twirling, panty-less, on random suspect bar stools or failing to use the toilet seat covers so helpfully provided in public restrooms. "Who knows?" I benignly replied, and we spent the rest of the trip in silence, each of us likely envisioning possible scenarios.
- A representative from the homeowners' association pounded on my front door one evening at dusk. I had heard the screened-porch

door squeal but hoped to avoid having to actually answer the front door to see who was standing inside the porch. Dressed in a bathrobe and currently in the midst of a pity party, I was in no mood to deal with what inevitably would be a complaint about the way I maintained (or failed to maintain) my condo's exterior. I pulled open the door to a rather surprised gentleman with a clipboard—he likely knew from experience or had heard from neighbors that I seldom answer the door or even am at home when anyone stops by. He proceeded to ask me about my windows and whether I would mind if a new neighbor installed frames a lighter color than mine, because my condo would now stand out as the only one in the block with older, darker frames and, to meet HOA standards, all window frames eventually should be the same color. He explained that my outdated frames could remain, as long as they still looked good, but, at some point, the change in my neighbor's frame color would require me to install light frames, too, because the balance of light versus dark frames in the community had now tipped to light. I said, rather bluntly, that I didn't care what color window frames anyone installed. The gentleman persisted, reminding me that my decision would have an impact not only on whether my new neighbor could have that color but my choice when I renovate my windows. I testily replied that I wasn't feeling well and, indeed, had terminal cancer and hoped I wouldn't have to install new windows or frames in the remainder of my lifetime. The gentleman hastily took a step back. "Oh! I see. Well, what kind of cancer do you have?" (as if that would make a difference either to my longevity or willingness to update my window frames). "Rec-tal," I enunciated with a hard c and sharp t, no doubt giving him an abhorrent mental image of the horrors hidden beneath my ratty robe. I have never seen anyone back out a screened-porch door so fast. The gentleman hesitantly stood just beyond the porch, as if distance and his clipboard would protect him from any free-roaming rectal cancer cells. He jotted down my response on his clipboard, mumbled an apology, and fled. Right then I learned the strategic power of turning "rec-tal" into a two-syllable weapon.

• While waiting for Jen to arrive for one of my chemo treatments, I sat numbly in the oncologist's waiting room. I hated chemo days to the point that I developed a physical reaction even to entering the door and signing in, and Jen always provided a nurturing presence on these stressful days. As I stared straight ahead and attempted to astral project myself anywhere else, a woman about my age tried to engage me in, as might be expected in an oncologist's office, cancer conversation. She was waiting with her sister, who had just been called away to have her vitals taken. "She has colon cancer. What's yours?" the woman asked casually and then smiled encouragingly. My weaponized "rec-tal" didn't put her off. (I have since perfected its strategic use.) "Oh," she perked up. "That's what killed Farrah Fawcett, isn't it? Wow, you have the same kind of cancer she had. I saw her documentary filmed while she was dying. It was really powerful." I nodded. Happily for me, Jen arrived, and I could shift my attention without being rude. Still, I wondered if I should be pleased that, at last, the famous Farrah Fawcett and I had something in common. (Actually, even that link is tenuous. Fawcett had anal cancer.)

• One day while I determinedly revised a conference paper at Panera, one of my favorite go-to places to munch, sip, and work simultaneously for hours at a time, my brain received an urgent "bathroom" warning from my lower body, despite my having scarfed four Imodium with breakfast. I slammed shut my laptop (hoping no one would bother to disconnect it and cart it off to their car while I was indisposed) and grabbed my purse. It is difficult to jog around tables while clenching one's gluteus maximus, but my brain by then was expecting immediate engagement with my enemy colon and screaming, "Outcoming!" To my alarm, the door to the women's restroom was blocked with a yellow construction barrier. I rushed to the counter and begged to use the men's room, which possibly was occupied. The manager, who just happened to be behind the register (and the counter just happened to be free of customers), immediately understood my panic. She led me to the women's bathroom, opened the door, and told the plumber fixing the sink to get out for a few minutes. He left, and I rushed to the largest stall. Unfortunately, my timing was about 10 seconds off, and I spent the next few minutes cleaning up myself, then sanitizing and spraying the toilet. However, I was grateful for privacy and a working toilet until I could return to "normal" and resume writing in the dining room. As I packed up later that morning, I spied the manager and went over to thank her for her help. "I have cancer," I explained quietly, "and sometimes I can't control my body." "I have cancer, too," she admitted, "and I know what you mean." To outsiders not seeing my mad dash earlier, she and I looked "normal"—just two women doing their jobs. Only we know how different we are from most people, but, as this most helpful manager reminded me, we are far from unique.

The most difficult expectations to deal with are often those from Heather, who grew up in what she terms a "sick house" where first her mother suffered kidney disease and, when Heather was a kindergartner, had a kidney transplant. That surgery substantially improved Nancy's quality of life, but she still must vigilantly monitor her health. When Heather was in high school, her father was diagnosed with multiple sclerosis. Bart already had had a heart attack and required bypass surgery, and his heart disease would continue to worsen for the rest of his life. When Heather was in her 20s, Bart was diagnosed with colon cancer, took chemo and had surgeries, and seemed to recover—for a little more than a year. He then "felt something was wrong," and he was right. The cancer had metastasized to his liver, among other places, and he was told he had about 18 months to live—if he agreed to chemo and exploratory surgeries to possibly prolong his life. All Heather's grandparents had already passed away before she became an adult. Dad quickly succumbed to lung cancer and died when Heather was two. Mom had a fatal heart attack en route home after Christmas with Bart, Nancy, and Heather; she missed Heather's high school graduation by about five months. Therefore, it isn't surprising that my diagnosis angered Heather—just as her father's had a few years earlier. It was unfair for either of us to die earlier than expected, especially of cancer. Even if either she or I had outgrown my being the "cool" aunt, she expected me to be around for her and her children for a long time.

When we finally discussed my continued longevity in September 2018, after she traveled without Nancy or her children to Daytona Beach to take care of some family business, she felt angry at the doctors who told me I was terminal. I had gone back to work. I still looked healthy and, during that trip, enjoyed taking her to our favorite beachside restaurants. In fact, I looked just the same as when she saw me in May, during the time when I encouraged visitors to hurry to Florida to see me before

I looked unrecognizably "bad." Heather confessed that she thought it was cruel for my oncologist to tell me in January that I had six months to live, when, in September, I was still going strong. Even the "possibly a year, on the outside" prognosis was being proven incorrect. I inadvertently perpetuated the cruelty by immediately sharing the bad news with my family. Heather felt angry that the doctors' news to me, and then mine to her, had caused us all so much anguish. Her expectation was that a terminal diagnosis with a prognosis of six months or slightly longer could be believed; my friends, my employer, and even I, who wants to live a long life, shared that expectation. After all, Dad's and Bart's prognoses were accurate within a few weeks. Although I am sure that Heather is happy that I was still around in September, she also mourned the loss of innocence—of assuming that my cancer had not come back after surgeries and treatments—and now must live again with the fear of impending loss. She, like so many of us, expected that technology and the doctors who interpret medical science for us would be much closer in an accurate estimate of my lifespan.

Whereas Heather's emotional response to my prognosis follows closely the stages of grief, others' expectations focus on a specific aspect of my life or, indeed, expectations for terminal cancer patients in general. Because warped humor and enjoyment of music tends to get me through the toughest times regarding cancer, I defer to world-famous deejay Casey Kasem for a way to introduce the Top 5 Countdown of Expectations for and by Those Dying of Cancer. (This style of introduction also harkens to my very brief time as a deejay in Ohio during the late 1970s and early 1980s.) Kasem's American Top 40 countdown was a staple of my weekend radio entertainment during the 1970s. Even in 2019, my Sunday drive is often punctuated with a rerun of Kasem's countdown from more than 30 years earlier. Anyone following my car on a Sunday coffee run may see me bopping to Peaches & Herb's "Shake Your Groove Thing" (1978) or emoting along with Barry Manilow on "Weekend in New England" (1976). As a result of Kasem's pop cultural influence on my high school and undergraduate college years, here are my Top 5 great expectations, beginning with number 5 and counting down to the Number 1 favorite across the country this week.

Starting off the countdown is an admonition against staying in one place and a tribute to all those great travel songs of the 20th century.

The older I become, the more I not only listen to but hear the power of the Monkees' Mickey Dolenz asking what he's doing "hangin' 'round." Dolenz may have agonized about getting on the "Last Train to Clarksville" (1966), but I agree that I, too, should be on the nearest form of transportation—train, plane, automobile. However, the Number 5 spot on the great expectations countdown usually leads to a plaintive warning from surgeons and concerned family members that contradicts Dolenz's musical wisdom. That's right, Number 5 is the popular refrain

5. I cannot/should not travel alone.

Surgeons have explained that, because of my numerous DVTs and PEs while I underwent chemotherapy, I am at a greater risk for blood clots when my circulation is compromised, such as on a long-distance flight or drive. As my compromise, I wear knee-high compression socks that promote circulation. During a long-haul flight, I attempt to stretch as often as possible, given the realities of being seat-belted for hours at a time without the opportunity to get up. I'm not nearly as careful about drinking lots of water, mostly because the more I am hydrated, the more likely my bowels will speed up digestion or use all that cleansing liquid to enjoy even more (and more unexpected) movements. When I travel, I worry about rushing to a restroom up to 20 times a day on "bad days" or around eight to 10 on "good days." (In grosser terms, friends have joked that on bad days I am "crappy" but even on good days I'm "full of shit.") Thus, I can understand the medical concern over my traveling alone even while I feel healthy.

The longer I survive post-death notice, the more likely I am to need a companion, beyond the enjoyment of sharing my on-the-road experiences. Already I rely on Jen to help with baggage check-in at the airport. On board, she either graciously slides into the center seat or springs up without question when I need to get to the aisle. She blissfully ignores how many times I excuse myself or makes no comment if I nibble a few bites—or skip a meal entirely—because I'm afraid to eat more. She brings "supplies" (my code word for more diapers, wipes, and plastic bags) when my purse has been left too far away or I've run out of clean clothes.

The problem comes with the difference between having a friend to share toothpaste with and requiring a caregiver to give me medication and wheel me from place to place. During my friendship with Jen, she has been both at different stages of my illness. However, I feel much less guilt and anxiety over being a burden when I can literally and figuratively carry my weight on a trip.

Beyond the physical difficulties that may make travel more proscribed and carefully planned as I decline are the normal reasons why a senior woman shouldn't travel alone: age, decreased ability to defend herself physically, and loneliness. Although these factors vary greatly from person to person (not just senior woman to senior woman), they seem to form the rationale for everything from public scrutiny to pity to ridicule to condemnation, depending upon how egregious others think this social transgression may be. "It just isn't done," a former teacher, well into her 80s, explained gently when I became a solo traveler in my 40s. Mom was more direct: "You can't do that anymore," she firmly told me after I spent a month getting to know New Zealand, variously on my own, with a new friend, or as part of a small tour group. On an afternoon a few months later, when Mom and Aunt Bettye reminisced about high school, my aunt mused, "We never even raised our hand in class." I had just shared a story about another adventure, which included taking a train into Edinburgh and talking to actors at the film festival; as a long-time Billy Boyd fan, I was thrilled to talk with him on the red carpet and in the lobby after a screening. Chatting with Thomas Carlyle, then probably best known for *Trainspotting* (1996) or *The Full Monty* (1997), was an unexpected plus. Such name dropping often seemed egoistic and embarrassing for those who didn't want others to judge me harshly for being so self-involved. "*We* didn't want to be noticed," Mom added. "We never wanted to stand out and do things like you do."

I believe their solidarity regarding being as inconspicuous as possible resulted from the way many (most?) women were reared in the 1930s and early 1940s. Also, because widowed Mom-Ma Margie struggled to bring up a son and five daughters on her husband's small pension and her occasional work as a school bus driver, she didn't want outsiders to closely scrutinize her family. If they didn't do anything to draw attention to themselves, she was more likely to keep her family together. Mom's and Aunt Bettye's admonition wasn't meant to be malicious or excluding but to remind me of the unwritten familial and social rules that single women are asking for trouble if they stand out in class, much less travel alone, and I admit that any single traveler needs to be aware of potential dangers. However, that doesn't mean that they—or I—should stay safely at home. Nonetheless, being terminally ill only exacerbates others' concern.

In the early 1990s, when my parents stayed with Bart, Nancy, and toddler Heather at their just-outside-Wooster, Ohio, home, which, at the time, was on a long, quiet road in the country, Dad wanted to build up his strength by walking. He was about halfway through the time span physicians had given him for living with fast-growing, metastasizing lung tumors, and he had been taking tests at the Cleveland Clinic. During one visit, he bragged to the doctor that he liked to walk alone nearly a mile down the gravel road before he turned around to come back, usually while Bart and Nancy were away at work and Mom stayed behind with her own health issues. The doctor tried gently telling Dad that perhaps Mom could drive him down the road a mile and then follow him in the car as he walked back to the house. Dad stubbornly shook his head; he was an "I'll do it my way" kind of guy. Finally, the doctor starkly explained that Dad might be able to go down the road but someday soon would collapse on the way back and (in the pre-mobile phone days) not be able to get help. He would be stuck and could die before someone found him. Taking that solo walk (i.e., traveling alone, even a mile) was not worth the immediate risk of dying. Truly my father's daughter, I expect that it will take that kind of warning (or a close call) before I accept that I can't travel alone—or travel at all.

Back on our countdown, coming in at Number 4 is a happy-go-lucky little number that suggests how the world should operate, not necessarily how it does. In 1966, Lesley Gore had a hit single, "Sunshine, Lollipops, and Rainbows," from the previous year's movie *Ski Party*, but who composed that optimistic little ditty that debuted on Gore's *Mixed-Up Hearts* album? The answer—when I return (following a suitable commercial break for Depends).

Did you guess the composer who went on to record the Oscar-winning soundtrack to *The Way We Were* (1973) and the Tony-winning Broadway musical *A Chorus Line*? The answer, of course, is Marvin Hamlisch (who happens to be another of my all-time favorite composers and musicians. I played the introductory-level piano sheet music to most of his movie or Broadway themes throughout the 1960s and 1970s). "Sunshine, Lollipops, and Rainbows" extols the virtues of being in love, but one line can easily be co-opted to fit this item on my countdown. It describes how everything "wonderful" is certain to come along simply by the virtue of one's state of being—in Gore's case, being in love; in mine, being nearer death. According to such widely divergent people in my life as my niece and my ophthalmologist,

4. I should automatically be granted perks (i.e., something "wonderful") because I'm terminal.

After Heather drove her two preschool children and Nancy to visit me in Florida in May 2018, we all stayed together in a rented condo on the beach at Ponce Inlet. (It rained constantly that week—a weather phenomenon that has not occurred before or since. So much for the beach or Disney World being the happiest place on earth for a very disappointed me.) Nevertheless, I hope the children, at least, have some pleasant memories of meeting Mickey or running into and out of the waves between thunderstorms.

While Heather and I were making a dinner run down the road to Señor Taco one evening, she commented that it was great that this vacation didn't cost me anything. I asked her what she meant. "Well, because you have cancer," she said. I assured her that, although I was extremely thrilled to have a "friend" discount from the condo's owner, I still paid for our week's stay, as well as the Disney World tickets and overnights on park property. Heather was indignant. "They should give that to you!" Perhaps she was thinking of the Make-a-Wish Foundation or similar groups who strive to make the wish of a terminally ill child (most often) or adult (occasionally) come true, without any cost to the family. I'm fortunate to be able to make my wishes of vacations for family or friends and me come true while I'm still recognizable as the vibrant woman they knew, but I was startled to realize that Heather—and likely many others—think that cancer at least provides special financial perks in the way of free vacations.

However, I do admit that cancer has occasionally provided perks for me when I've been wheelchair-bound and too weak to walk more than a step or two. During a trip to Universal Studios in the midst of my chemo treatments in 2016, Jen and Joy took turns pushing me around the park. I asked about getting a go-to-the-head-of-the-line-first pass when we visited Guest Services, where I pathetically pleaded that I needed such a pass because I was undergoing chemo and couldn't stand, in line or anywhere else. The representative assured me that, if I was rolled up to a ride, the attendant would ensure that I got on. Probably I should have been ashamed of my glee, but I was remorseless (and relentless in pursuing ride after ride). Joy or Jen rolled me to the first ride host we saw at each attraction, and we were led through back hallways or up lifts until I was inches away from a ride. Apparently not too many rolling cancer patients were in the queue ahead of us that day, because, after a wait of five minutes or less, I was strapped into a car for our first ride through Harry Potter's world—and so our day went, from ride to ride, wheelchair to belted metal seat and back. On the way home, I joked that I would've gotten cancer sooner if I had known I could go to the head of the line every time. So, yes, occasionally there are perks with cancer—but not nearly enough of the financially beneficial ones to suit everyone who hears of my plight.

My ophthalmologist, with whom I have swapped travel stories and recommendations, was taken aback when he learned that, a year after my terminal diagnosis, I returned to teaching. Of course, that semester I received two course releases—one in order to continue editing a journal, the other in order to write two books. However, the "release" was from teaching, not from an equivalent number of work hours. I also taught one student in a senior thesis course, as well as a full class—23 students—in an introductory speech course. This load is very light, and I greatly appreciated the thoughtfully prepared schedule that allowed me to work on campus two days a week and from home the rest of the time. Nonetheless, the schedule was still challenging some days when I felt bad or my incontinence proved to be an insurmountable problem to staying in the classroom. Even after learning about these blessed accommodations to my condition, my ophthalmologist leaned back in surprise and crossed his arms in complaint. "I needed the medical insurance," I explained, after detailing how kindly the faculty and administrators in my department and college were treating me. They made it possible for me to work a full-time schedule, resulting in a full paycheck and benefits. No matter how much I enjoy being part of a university faculty, having cancer has reset my priorities, and working 12- or 14-hour days is no longer my marker for success. However, I expressed my worry about what would happen if I live past the next academic year's scheduled sabbatical, which provides full benefits and half salary. I confided that I didn't think I could return to teaching four classes, my course releases having been used up by that point. "I think they should just give you the benefits," he protested. "You've worked there nearly 20 years." Because we have always made dark jokes about my life expectancy, we teased that, after all, my employers wouldn't have to pay for benefits very long.

The expectation that anyone—from theme park operations or employers to individual friends or well-wishers—automatically will provide freebies to the terminally ill is one that mostly goes unfulfilled. That's not to say that people haven't generously donated time or money to help me travel or be able to work at home—they have, and I am grateful. However, cancer is not a warped fairy godmother who turns a giant tumor into a gilded carriage for a weekend on the town.

Returning to our countdown, I have to mention religion or spirituality, which, on many of my friends' and family members' Top 5 list regarding anything in life, is always right at the top. Number 3 on my expectations countdown belongs to the Bosco Boys and their 2015 song, "Who Says You Can't Be a Saint." An urban dictionary definition of the lower-cased term *bosco boys* references home turf Don Bosco Prep High School in Ramsey, New Jersey, as the origin of the name. A bosco boy is kind, fun loving, loyal, and full of school spirit. The singing duo Bosco Boys also believe in Spirit—Steve DeMaio and Steve Eguino studied to become Catholic priests with the Salesians of Don Bosco (St. Benedict Parish). Their lyrics emphasize the goodness in everyday activities— including teaching and being a mom (or, I suppose, an auntie)—and suggest that we keep doing our duties to the best of our ability. The repeated refrain provides the assurance that God will work through each of us if we continue to find holiness in everyday tasks. Number 3 reflects the way that life should be lived if one is going to be more Godlike as well as God-fearing:

3. I should be more saintly or inspirational because my time is short.

The expectation that I automatically will become a better person as a result of disease is ranked lower on my list of Top 5 expectations partly because I'm more secular than traditionally religious. I'm not a martyr for cancer, and just because my illness is terminal doesn't automatically make me a better person—or even someone who goes out of her way to try to be a better person. If I'm inspirational to others, I'm glad to have inadvertently served that role, but my aim every day isn't to be a source of inspiration. Nonetheless, I agree with the Bosco Boys' attitude toward sainthood and agree that it's reasonable that I do my duties well and as pleasantly as possible. However, I always tried to meet that criterion, even without the possibility of my work being part of a saintly path.

I received a message similar to that in the Bosco Boys' song from the kindly gentleman who prints the journal I edited, *Studies in Popular Culture*. We had only emailed each other a few times a year, mostly about the number of copies to be printed and the publication timeline. When I finally let him know that a new editor would take over beginning with the next issue, I explained that my cancer had returned. Two years earlier, when I emailed him that no cancer cells had been detected in my post-chemo scans, he had rejoiced and thanked God. Thus, it was difficult for me to update him with the news that the cancer metastasized and was untreatable. He responded with an inspiring message, reminding me that God is not done with me yet and obviously has something left for me to do. Without adhering to the tenets of a specific religion, I believe that my friend is right—I have a purpose (more than being someone with cancer) and intend to keep doing my work and being as involved as possible with loved ones as long as I can.

Number 2 on my countdown of Top 5 expectations is a variation on this theme:

2. My spiritual beliefs and practices are not sufficient to save me.

Going all the way back to 1979, here's Stevie Wonder with "Superstition." Among *Billboard*'s own countdown of Wonder's top Hot 100 hits throughout his career, "Superstition" comes in at Number 10. On January 22, 1977, it hit Number 1 on the Hot 100 (Corpuz). Key lyrics warn against believing in things that people cannot (or should not) understand, because they can invite the devil's presence. Superstition, Wonder insists, is not the way to go, especially if you're preparing to be gone.

Many people in my life are what I call traditionally religious. They, like I once did, attend church regularly, read the Bible, pray, and try to do good. They may accept that I've had trouble with organized religion in my adult life because my beliefs may contradict part of a church's doctrine, especially when discussion turns to feminism or LGBTQIA+ rights. We may disagree, but, once I received a terminal diagnosis, they became more actively concerned that my spiritual beliefs will not save me from damnation. Assuaging their anxiety about my soul after death is difficult because my ideas seem to others to be based on superstition, not faith. Throughout my life, I have attended religious services with friends or colleagues from a wide range of religions, and I find something to admire and emulate in each. The final word for me is that I am comforted by my spiritual beliefs, although they differ probably from everyone else's.

Some people may think I'm trying to hedge my bets regarding an afterlife through my multicultural approach to spirituality. I was baptized in the United Methodist Church and was confirmed as a teenager. I believe the teachings of Jesus are valid ways to live one's life because they affirm that I should love others, treat them as I wish to be treated, and act on that love by helping out in whatever way possible. I also find value in the teachings of the Buddha, but I am not Buddhist. I am not a born-into member of many cultures and societies whose teachings about harmony and balance make sense to me. Because Mom was interested in Edgar Cayce and read books by and about him, so did I. Over the years I have participated in shamanic workshops, had psychic readings, and practiced Reiki and yoga. All of these activities fed into my spirituality, but I have never felt that they make me less grateful to a divine being.

Therefore, my travels since my cancer diagnosis have led me to pray in cathedrals around the United States and other countries. One Thursday afternoon in London, at the Anglican St. Martin-in-the-Field, I felt my spirit rise with the music from a quartet playing Medieval liturgical music; that, to me, was a highly religious experience. When I visited New Mexico in July, I heard of El Sanctuario de Chimayo Shrine. Following a winding road from Taos and a spotty GPS signal, I visited the Shrine, where I meditated in the chapel, bought plastic containers from nearby shops, and filled them with holy dirt to take home. In the past few months, I've received Reiki-infused massages at spa resorts, been prayed over at a car dealership when someone overheard that I didn't feel well, been gifted with Bibles, and been sent healing energy. Every day I express my gratitude for life, mine and the lives of so many people who wish me well. For me, this amalgam of practices helps me express my belief that love and harmony are universally recognized spiritual concepts that can help heal. Others may find my actions desperate, a blind groping for making meaning of my impending death or grasping for a cure. Yet, that's not my motivation or reality. I am at peace with my beliefs, which is the important part.

Perhaps my collection of beliefs might be another sign to family or friends that I'm mentally incapacitated. A few have suggested as much. Next up on our countdown is an oldie but goodie written by Willie Nelson that just might replace "On the Road Again" as my theme song. Although Nelson has recorded the country classic "Crazy" several times, including as a duet with Elvis Costello or Diana Krall, perhaps the best-known version goes back to 1962, just a year after Nelson wrote this legendary ballad. Who took "Crazy" to Number 2 on the country chart in 1962? The answer—in 60 seconds. (Play a 60-second spot for Imodium.)

OK, this was an easy one. Who took "Crazy" near the top of the country chart for 21 weeks in 1962—and whose version is immortalized on *Rolling Stone*'s The Greatest Songs of All Time, coming in at Number 85? If you answered Patsy Cline, you're correct. Although many memorable recordings of "Crazy" have graced the charts over the years, Cline first made it a hit. She captured the anguish of losing, in her case, love (in mine, credibility) and berates herself for being crazy to think her relationship could have led to anything but this sad separation. The inevitability of loss resonates with those close to someone with cancer who believe that the terminally ill person's mood changes, sentimentality, or everyday mistakes or misunderstandings are the unavoidable result of chemotherapy. This variation of "Crazy" tops my countdown of great expectations:

1. I am crazy because of chemo.

Proving I am not mentally deficient after months of IV chemotherapy is difficult, because so many people know of loved ones who became cruel, violent, hallucinatory, or irrational near the end of life. Even if cancer has metastasized in the brain, family caregivers may still attribute this physical cause of lapses in logic or mood swings to medication. Of course, some types of medications can have side effects, as Bart found out when he hallucinated a lovely herd of deer running through the backyard. However, even without further metastasis, side effects to medications, or mood changes as part of grief or pain, "dead" people like me may still have to fight a surprisingly common expectation that chemo has irreparably damaged rationality.

When I watched the *Victoria* television episode "A Show of Unity" in early 2019, I empathized with Queen Victoria (Jenna Coleman) and her young son, Prince Bertie (Laurie Shepherd). Scientifically minded Prince Albert (Tom Hughes) comes to believe that both Victoria and Bertie are hereditarily limited in their ability to think. After learning more about the then-popular study of phrenology, Albert becomes convinced that science proves that Victoria's temper is irrational and Bertie is too weak minded to understand the logic behind chess. No matter what Victoria says, she cannot convince Albert, once he has heard the "science" behind his conviction, that she is a rational woman or their son can understand abstract concepts.

Similarly, I have teasingly been referred to as "cra-cra" when I confess that I don't understand some fine points of interpersonal relationships or reasons why (to my mind—which becomes part of the argument against me) a perfectly innocent comment or action set off a loved one's intense emotional reaction. I've been told that I misinterpret or miss interpersonal cues, but being unable to relate to people is not really my fault because "chemo makes you crazy." According to this argument, my interpretation of reality is skewed because of treatments taken a few years earlier, and nothing I can do can convince others that I am as mentally sound now as I was pre-cancer. If I'm angry or defensive, any raw emotion can be condescendingly explained away with "You've had chemo; no wonder you're not thinking straight." When I express my desire to live at home until death—although I recognize that I will require hospice assistance at least—my wish is dismissed as unrealistic because I live alone and have no husband or children to care for me. Expecting that anyone who has taken chemotherapy is automatically unstable or incapable of rational thought seems unfair—but, then, I must be crazy.

My Top 5 list of great expectations may differ from that of other "dead" people, but I bet we've heard a lot of similar expectations or had them ourselves. Even advice by psychologists or other medical experts still may irritate those of us who appreciate their good intentions. An article from the Certified Nursing Academy (CNA) provides the following guidance to future health-care workers dealing with the terminally ill: "Don't tell patients to eat healthier, meditate, or maintain an optimistic attitude. They may decide to do these things, but don't force them. They probably already feel guilty or defeated and don't need to be reminded of their shortcomings or what may have caused their condition."

At least for now, I can speak up for myself if I don't want to do something (such as eat when I am going to be away from home for hours afterward) or, more likely, specifically want to do something (such as attempt a movie marathon at a local cinema). However, the last part of the CNA's rationale is flawed in my case: I don't feel guilty or defeated. Depending on the day and my mood, my negative emotions may involve feeling tired, anxious, or envious of my former self. Yet, I don't take responsibility for having cancer. I don't know that, even if I had been a heavy smoker, I would feel guilty that cancerous cells metastasized in my lungs. (I never smoked beyond one ill-fated attempt.) Although some family members have suggested that ingesting the charcoaled steaks Dad so lovingly grilled on Sunday afternoons during my 20s led to Bart's or my colorectal cancer, none of us ever heard of polycyclic aromatic hydrocarbons and their possible link with cancer. Instead, I have fond memories of our backyard picnics, the foodie highlight being a medium-well T-bone, its juices sizzling on my plate.

As the CNA posits, I may someday feel defeated. If I could live another decade or two healthfully, I would. To this point, I'm not defeated in my day-to-day life. I will always want more of the good stuff but am satisfied with my successes, pleasures, and experiences. If I agree with any of that last part of the CNA statement, it is that I admit that I have shortcomings that may have affected my longevity. If I had chosen a different medical team or a different hospital, would my surgery have taken place sooner or more successfully removed the rogue cancer cells that had grown outside my bowel and, eventually, set up shop in my lungs? If I had decided to stick with the stronger type of chemo that was increasing my neuropathy and affecting my breathing, would any post-surgery cancer cells have been destroyed? If I had searched for second, third, fourth opinions, especially out of state, would I have found the winning combination of facility and facilitators to eliminate the cancer? I don't know. I followed the best advice I received at the time but wasn't terribly proactive in seeking a wide range of options. Nonetheless, I accept "it is what it is"—I can't go back in time, no matter how many *Time Tunnel*, *Quantum Leap*, or *Doctor Who* episodes I watch. I can only decide not to beat myself up that my judgment may not have been what others' would have been in the same situation.

When I see friends or colleagues once diagnosed with cancer but who today are living cancer free, I am happy for them—but I can't be angry at myself for not having the same outcome. One morning, as Jen and I prepared for a day at a conference, I told Jen of a recent conversation with a mutual acquaintance who had recently received a cancer diagnosis. I chuckled as I noted that every time we talked, she stated that her cancer is curable and, once treatments and surgery are over, she'll be fine. I recounted to Jen that, out of all the people we know professionally who have been treated for cancer in the past three years, I'm the only one to score highly on CEA results and go terminal. Using a descriptor familiar to teachers and students, I groused, "I'm such a curve killer." Jen laughed with me. "That's funny," she said. "Add that to your memoir."

If I look at longevity another way, one that allows me to score highest on number of days I have been alive, I also am a curve killer for my family. I have outlived Dad and Bart and enjoyed at least a "bonus year" after a terminal diagnosis. I hope that they would have been happy that I outlived my initial prognosis, not envious or regretful that I lived longer than they. Longevity, like cancer stage or status, shouldn't become a competition. No one wins in a game of "my cancer is better/worse" than yours.

In 1984, what would be the first edition of Heidi Murkoff's *What to Expect When You're Expecting* was published. It has since gone on to multiple editions in multiple formats, including film. Although the book has been updated several times, it provides a primer that explains and illustrates the typical progression of a normal pregnancy. If only cancer—or even a specific kind of cancer, such as colorectal cancer—could have such a reputable guidebook (*What to Expect When You're Terminal*, maybe? How about *What to Expect When You're Expecting Imminent*

Cancer Death?). Instead, most people rely on their oncologists' or surgeons' understanding of a typical disease progression and standard methods of treatment. Because I defied my oncologist's expectations for more than a year, and the standard treatment didn't work for me (which, possibly, is why the cancer metastasized and, along the way, I have had additional physical problems), I especially relied on common expectations for cancer patients to anticipate what would happen next. As the stories in this memoir illustrate, expecting the unexpected may be part of many people's cancer journeys.

No one—not even I, writing a book that I hope will help others faced with cancer—can understand exactly what someone else who is terminally ill with cancer is going through. Effective, frequent communication is the only way to get others to understand how I feel right now or what worries me about the future. I prefer to be direct or even blunt because subtle conversational cues often elude me, and neither loved ones nor medical professionals may correctly understand how or what I am feeling. As a culture, stating our expectations and sharing aloud our hopes and fears about living and dying with cancer are the only ways we can eliminate the stigma of cancer and stop replaying my—and others'—Greatest Hits countdown of Great (or Not-So-Great) Expectations.

CHAPTER 10

Gratitude More Than Grief

Defying Expectations

Seneca wisely noted, "How late it is to begin really to live just when life must end! How stupid to forget our mortality, and put off sensible plans to our fiftieth and sixtieth years, aiming to begin life from a point at which few have arrived!" ("Seneca on the Shortness of Life"). Like Seneca (although I'm not nearly as wise in other matters), I learned from others' experiences.

Dad and I shared a strong work ethic, but I probably have enjoyed my many jobs far more than he did. However, I also avoided leadership roles, whereas he rose from insurance salesman to office manager to regional district manager at Western-Southern Life. Until I was around 12 or 13, Dad often worked evenings, and, because I was in school, I missed his brief afternoon visits at home, when he talked with Mom, dropped off his paycheck, or took a power nap before heading back to work. After all, we understood that he could sell more insurance policies to clients after they returned home from work after five. Mom was the one to attend the evening band concerts and school-day academic awards ceremonies.

Nevertheless, Dad always found ways to spend time with us, even when he frequently worked overtime. When Bart and I were very young, about three and six, respectively, Dad sometimes had to go into the office on Saturdays to finish paperwork. When Bart and I accompanied him, we were allowed to "play" with the large calculating machine, gleefully pushing buttons and pulling the lever to print columns of numbers. When that became too wasteful and annoying, Dad pulled safety-themed coloring books from the supply closet, and Bart and I colored

Sparky the Fire Dog as he warned us not to overload electrical sockets. We looked forward to Dad's overtime as playtime in a strange new environment. Afterward, Dad often took us fishing at Mr. Hollencamp's little lake behind his house. ("Hollie" worked for Dad and treated Bart and me as surrogate grandchildren.) Although baiting our hooks with worms or dough balls was probably as much work for Dad as filing accounts in the office, Bart and I enjoyed these Saturdays. Seated on the bank, cane poles in our hands, we quietly watched and waited for the red-and-white bobber to dip below the lake, then squealed when we hauled in a bluegill. Most of the time, Dad released our catch, but sometimes we caught large enough fish to be cleaned and fried for supper.

Balancing work with play became ingrained from these early memories, but so, too, was Dad's firm belief that one can only play after chores are done. Unfortunately, as I grew older, the number of "chores" tended to pile up, and I began to enjoy my consulting jobs as a trainer, technical writer, and editor more than socializing. For much of the time I was tenured at the University of Findlay, my days "off" from teaching were spent driving to a business or factory somewhere in Ohio to present a communication workshop or to gather information for writing a training manual. Work weeks of 60 to 70 hours were not uncommon, and, even when I was tired, I was pleased to have money in the bank and was satisfied with my professional expertise.

Despite the heavy work load, I still drove to nearby towns where Bart, then married to Nancy, worked as a journalist. As an entertainment editor for local newspapers, he sometimes needed someone to ride a camel or crawl into a hot air balloon and rise to the three-story limit of the tether, for example. I usually volunteered to be the guest in the photo he took to accompany his article. Later, Bart wrote newsletters for the Prairie Peddler Festival, held twice a year in the rolling hills of east-central Ohio, near Butler. The festival grounds steered crowds of visitors through rows of faux-Western booths where vendors, dressed in 19th-century work clothes, demonstrated skills like making beeswax candles or playing dulcimers. Crafts of all types were on display, but this version of the Old West also featured a jail and an outlaw gang's hideout. Bart became Doc Laborday (a play on Doc Holiday), one of the colorful characters wandering the festival and, a few times a day, engaging and attempting to evade the Sheriff, who sometimes locked up Doc Laborday's gang in the makeshift jail. Of course, they soon managed to escape (and hilarity ensued). Other times, the Sheriff let the gang retreat to their hideout at the back of the property. Bart created a character for me, the Modern Dance Kid, and for a few seasons we were playmates at Prairie Peddler. These weekends made my life special, and Bart presented me with opportunities to enjoy being with him, Nancy, and Heather. Work didn't seem overwhelming when I looked forward to spending time with my "little" brother.

When I had earned my Ph.D. and become employed (twice) in tenurable university positions, I skillfully blended work and play. I flew to academic conferences to pitch ideas for books, pass around business cards to expand my network of contacts, and make presentations—but, between and around these intensive work experiences, I took day trips to admire the local scenery or have a new experience. During two separate Seattle conferences, I explored Mount Rainier. During a New York City convention of English teachers, I worked by day and haunted theatres by night. After receiving an award at a Dallas conference, Mom and I visited Aunt Bonnie and Janet, who lived "nearby," in Texas terms. I spent all of one sabbatical in New Zealand, conducting research at a film institute in Wellington and on "Hobbit" tours around the country. Even before starting a tour of the Netherlands, Belgium, Germany, and Luxembourg—supposedly a true summer vacation—I arrived in Amsterdam two days early so I could conduct research at the Van Gogh Museum for a book I was writing about Vincent's imposing presence in popular culture.

All this work-play balance resulted from Dad's early influence on my perception of how the world works—and he never implied that I couldn't achieve what I wanted just because I'm female. His early death also became a lesson on how to live. When Dad was barely 60 (and I was 36), he was suddenly diagnosed with terminal lung cancer and died a little more than three months later. Only a few months before he was diagnosed, he retired early so that he and Mom could live their dream life on a Florida lake.

The suddenness of his loss—and our loss of him—confirmed my earlier education that, even amidst a heavy workload, one must have some fun. Vacations shouldn't be put off until retirement. From the time I was 36 until I was myself diagnosed with cancer at 58, I refused to teach during the summers, although I diligently wrote books and chapters for a variety of publishers and became a contributing editor for online magazine *PopMatters*. Whereas writing is certainly work, for me it is also a joy and often downright fun. Even during my illness, I have continued to write—or go to what my good friend Donna Barbie calls my "happy place"—but I also take time to go to the beach or an Orlando theme park to enjoy what most people consider "fun" activities. After my terminal diagnosis, I also became determined to be more social—to reconnect face to face with the family members and friends I usually caught up with online or on the phone. I invite people to visit me so we can have a good time in Florida together. At least once a month I share breakfast, afternoon tea, or a pub night with friends, and more frequently I tag along with my adoptive Wojton-Carney-Arias family on a kid-friendly adventure.

That's why I not only agree with Seneca's assessment of the shortness of life but, more important, enjoy the quality and variety of experiences I have had and will continue to wring from life until I can no longer breathe. I am my father's daughter, who learned from his life and death how to use the time allotted me.

This philosophy, however, hasn't always prepared me to deal with my expectations about dying. Even as I write this memoir, I am unexpectedly healthy enough to enjoy mornings of writing at Sweet Marlay's coffee shop, immersed in the homey environment and friendly patter. When I'm full of café au lait, the caffeine keeps my fingers flying across the keyboard. I don't know how bad "bad" will become or how quickly I will fulfill my oncologist's prognosis. All I can do is live today.

I watched a *60 Minutes* segment in which Senator John McCain, who had been diagnosed with terminal brain cancer, admitted, "I have feelings sometimes of fear of what happens. But as soon as I get that, I say … 'You've been around a long time, old man. You've had a great life. You've had a great experience'" ("One of a Kind"). I concur with this sentiment and approach to life. I feel relief at knowing what is happening and gratitude for having the resources and time to live the best life possible as long as possible now that I know. Although I seem to have skipped the majority of the stages of grief (denial, anger, bargaining, depression, acceptance ["The Five Stages of Grief"]) through my emphasis on gratitude for what I have had and still have, such an approach can seem to others like being stuck in denial or exhibiting an embarrassing naiveté.

Accepting that I have and am expected to die because of cancer is something I think about and deal with every day. I wake with the knowledge—but not the fear—of my mortality. My body is changing, but sometimes I can't tell if that is normal aging or more rapid deterioration because of disease. During an appointment with my oncologist in October 2018, when I was supposed to be already dead or in the latter stages of dying, he asked if I had noticed any changes to my breathing. I told him about my summer drive from Farmington to Taos, New Mexico. When I stopped along the way to climb hills or even stride up paved inclines, I quickly grew short of breath. I had the same problem walking uphill to overlooks at the Grand Canyon in September. "Am I having trouble because of less oxygen in higher elevations?" I asked, certain that my huff-puffing resulted from growing tumors and was exacerbated by thinner air. "No," he replied. "You're getting older." He tactfully didn't mention that I am out of shape; my "exercise" walks take place on flat beaches where I frequently stop to pick up shells or watch the pelicans.

Even my oncologist has been surprised that I persistently live months longer than predicted, an expectation I am gratified to have defied. His best advice is to "go live your life." I think Seneca would approve.

CHAPTER 11

The End Is Nigh

So far, I have thwarted my oncologist's expectations for my longevity, and I hope to follow his instruction to "live my life" for months to come. Yet, I live under the shadow of others' and my expectations. My and my loved ones' greatest expectation is that, because I have survived longer than expected, I will continue to do so and feel almost or as good as I feel on my best days, which seems in the typical range of health for a woman in her early 60s. The fantasy is that next year or the year after I will still be around just as vibrantly as I am now—that this "bonus year" as a "dead" woman sets the precedent for the remainder of my cancer journey.

However, cancer is unpredictable, and I have no guarantee that my robust health will continue or for how long. The hovering "not-so-great" expectations are the stuff of nightmares. They are the result of too much interwebs reading about death statistics and cancer patients' horror stories of pain and the death of hope. Based on my family's cancer experiences, I can't expect that mine will be much different, but I also have managed to be more optimistic about my future. (However, I haven't yet faced the pain of enlarged tumors and organ failure, so perhaps it's not fair to say that I will maintain a better mental outlook in the long term.) The familiar saying "Hope for the best; plan for the worst" seems to be a pragmatic approach, but I prefer motivational speaker Denis Waitley's advice to "expect the best, plan for the worst, and prepare to be surprised" (Meah).

Therefore, a roadmap to help me navigate current and future realities, as well as myriad expectations and their emotional tolls, is imperative to keeping me focused on my journey as I travel, instead of freaking out over what may take place before I reach my final destination. I plan milestones—whether business or leisure related—and head toward them with the confidence that I will arrive at the next planned destination. I must continue to live in a state of hopeful awareness and gratitude for every "bonus" day I live past a terminal diagnosis. Before the end, I likely will be house- or hospice-bound or will travel outside the confines of bed only in my mind, but, as Aragorn fiercely proclaims during his pre-battle motivational speech before the final onslaught in *The Lord of the Rings: The Return of the King* (2003): "Today is not that day!"

Although every day is special in some way, December holidays have always held deep personal meaning in addition to serving as calendar milestones. They remind me that the end is nigh and to prepare for it, reminisce about it, and celebrate a new beginning arising from an ending. Thus, throughout the December 2018 semester break and festive season, I became determined to experience the world as a social butterfly and to express my love for the people who share my life and have stuck around after my cancer diagnosis. I shared a trio of BJ's pazookis with Sophie Jorgensen, who has been a valuable assistant during my journal editorship (and a valued friend); sipped tea with Donna Barbie in various cafés; gossiped and brainstormed book ideas with Mike Perez over breakfast; shared a pub night with colleague and friend Sandy Branham; and savored high tea with Chas Mullins and Scott Stewart, whose friendship began through fandom but became deeper over the years. When I couldn't be physically near family or friends, we talked on the phone. My mobile phone was hot by the time Nancy and I finished our nearly two-hour conversation and caught up on everything happening in the Porter home. Since we were about 10 years old, Genie and I have wrapped each other's presents in Santa paper, and this year was no exception. Once we opened our gifts, she called me to thank me (and I her), and we compared holiday activities. Janet and I also can talk on the phone for hours, once we get going; we may talk infrequently but cover everything we've been doing or thinking since the last time we talked.

This year I also wanted to experience the festive season, both through recapturing glimpses of Christmases past and participating in Christmas present (and its presents). Alone, I walked down memory lane while strolling through an exuberant display of holiday lights and Christmas odes to fandoms (including Mickey Mouse, *Star Wars*, Charlie Brown and Snoopy, even dinosaurs and dragons); each year the owners of the Twi-Light II motel on U.S. 1 in Holly Hill gift the community with extravagant old-fashioned displays of lights and inflatable Christmas yard decorations set up on every available space on, around, and between the motel's little cabins. Twi-Light II's displays let me walk through time, past trees with large blue-and-white bulbs just like we had on the first Christmas trees I remember. Their inflatable scenes of Snoopy and the Red Baron or Charlie Brown and the Peanuts gang remind me of all the holiday specials Bart and I watched together as children and the funnies we read in every Sunday's newspaper. The Wojtons keep dragging me into the present when I'm in danger of getting lost in the past. With them, I marveled at the large-scale technology of holiday decorations on display at SeaWorld, where we visited the Christmas village and ooh-aahed over music-synchronized tree lights, and I snuck a bite of chocolate-covered bacon from Jen's and Layla's "dinner." Long before Christmas, I cherished my loved ones' gifts of time, love, and shared moments.

With Joy's and Carlos' combined families, I celebrated Christmas Eve in their Longwood home. Grandparents, children, and children's children first feasted; then the kids ran in and out of the house, working off their sugar high, while the grownups talked until it was time to open presents. During my Midwest Christmases, opening presents was a highly organized affair, with one person carefully untaping a gift while everyone else watched. The recipient thanked the giver, and everyone commented on whatever the gift turned out to be. When Heather was a toddler, she loved opening packages of new clothes. "Put on!" she insisted, and gift giving halted until Heather had tried on her new outfit. Because Heather usually received lots of pretty clothes, opening presents in the Porter household often lasted several hours. Not so at Joy and Carlos' Christmas celebration, as the generations of Ariases, Carneys, and Wojtons got down to business. After adults passed around the packages from beneath the tree, everyone opened everything at once. The joyful carnage as tinseled paper flew from boxes and eager hands plunged into gift bags reminded me of films of piranhas' feeding frenzy. Somehow everyone managed to show everyone else the just-opened treasures, say thank you, and immediately try on or try out the gift. In a very short time, the children returned to running around the house and yard, this time playing with new toys.

I enjoyed sharing the holiday with so many friends and family members, in person or over the phone. Nonetheless, I also enjoyed some "alone time" before New Year's Eve. I've always said that the two settings in which I feel most comfortable are bookstores and theatres. Despite my gradually increasing dependence on my phone (not only for practical reasons like summoning help but entertainment ones like reading fanfiction in airports), I prefer paper books; the heft of a book in my hand or purse, the satisfaction of turning pages and seeing how much I've read and how much is left to go, and the love expressed by well-worn covers are comforting. My early attachment to books (and the act of writing) and to the stories people tell make bookstores feel homey and welcoming. In December, I began reading a series of biographies or memoirs of famous people whose work I've enjoyed throughout my life: Sally Field, Olivia Hussey, Robin Williams, Roger Daltrey, Vincent van Gogh, Rembrandt. Once the semester's classes had ended, I often could be found sitting for hours in a café or bookshop, low-fat latte in front and to the right of a book propped on a table or arm of a chair. I equally love the theatre, and, although I've seen friends Chas Mullins and Libbie Searcy on stage in local productions, most often I travel to see touring companies in Orlando or fly off to New York, Toronto, or London to see multiple plays (or one play multiple times, if I've fallen in love with an actor or a performance). This December my trip to New York fell through, but I looked forward to returning to London to see Martin Freeman in Harold Pinter's *The Dumb Waiter*. A few months earlier, after a very difficult day, I impulsively bought tickets from the Pinter Theatre's website, figuring someone could get a refund for the trust if I wasn't around in February to see the play. In December, I finally committed to booking international flights and indulging in arranging for a car to pick me up at Gatwick and take me to my hotel in the city. Having something to look forward to, and feeling positive that I would be watching one of my favorite actors on stage only a few feet away, is an extravagant but highly motivating part of my "health plan."

Although live theatre is special, movie theatres also have been an important part of my life, ever since Mom first took me to see *Lady and the Tramp* (1955). During childhood, Bart and I often spent afternoons at the Ross in Evansville; I became engrossed with the cinematography of *Gone with the Wind* (1939), whereas he preferred *Planet of the Apes* marathons. Throughout our teens, summer wouldn't have been summer without at least a weekly visit to the Evansville or Sunset drive-ins for a double feature. Despite going to a cinema these days being much more of a production, I managed to catch up with holiday film releases and tried to see every Oscar-nominated movie.

On other on-my-own days, I drove up or down U.S. 1 toward a beach or an oceanfront restaurant for an early breakfast. After a foggy early morning drive to Flagler Beach, I breakfasted on Java Joint's deck. Through the shrouding mist, I watched lines of pelicans skim the waves in search of fish. On an even chillier morning, just after dawn I turned up at Sunglow Pier in Daytona Beach, where I watched the waves through the floorboards of Crabby Joe's while I munched my toast. Throughout the last week of the month and year, I walked along a lot of beaches, barely wetting my toes in the chilly water as I searched for shells. My December travels crisscrossed a 75-mile radius from my front door but racked up hundreds of miles on my car's odometer. On some days, when my body decided staying indoors was preferable, I embraced my inner Scrooge and sequestered myself at home with a mug of cocoa and a book. Even then, I refused to succumb to the ghosts of Christmas past or the specter of not living until Christmas future.

Perhaps because my condo is a short drive from the Atlantic, I enjoy beach-themed metaphors for relationships and life. In *Annie Hall* (1977), Alvy Singer (Woody Allen) agitatedly explains to Annie Hall (Diane Keaton) that a relationship is "like a shark…. It constantly has to move forward, or it dies." Although Alvy concluded that his relationship with Annie was a dead shark, I plan to keep moving forward—on my own two feet or wheeled along. As long as possible, my relationship with life will not become a dead shark.

In the past year I have joked to Jen and Chris (who wheeled me into movies, through zoos, and along hard-packed dirt paths at Highland Games when I was too weak from chemo to walk) that I want to be rolled to pool parties or the beach until I begin to decay, a la dead Bernie in *Weekend at Bernie's* (1989). In the movie, two men invited to the posh beach house of their boss, Bernie (Terry Kiser), need to drag around the body of their just-murdered host in order to keep enjoying the weekend getaway; they, as the film's Fandango plot synopsis explains, "decide not to let a little death spoil their vacation." My travel plans don't include giving up easily or foregoing the chance to get out of the house until I absolutely cannot move or be moved to enjoy an outing.

Nevertheless, sometimes I find myself withdrawing from a gathering of friends to watch them from the sidelines. I see them laughing and talking animatedly while children play around them. They make plans for going out together next weekend or next month. They look forward to doing the same things in the future, like going to an annual festival or returning to a favorite campsite same time, next year. This mental snapshot shows me what they will look like when I am gone. Life still goes on, and new friends and family members enter the picture. I'm reminded of hobbit Frodo's return to the Shire in Jackson's *The Lord of the Rings: The Return of the King* and, following an arduous journey to destroy the One Ring, his inability to be "normal" after what he had learned and had been through. Frodo/Elijah Wood asks in a voiceover, "How do you pick up the threads of an old life? How do you go on, when in your heart, you begin to understand, there is no going back?" In the past year, I have picked up and picked apart the threads of my pre-cancer life, and, although I have diligently tried to be as normal as possible, there is no going back to the woman I was.

The oft-quoted dialogue spoken by two notorious Southern belles in, respectively, *A Streetcar Named Desire* (1951) and *Gone with the Wind* (1939) preview what I envision as my future. (Both characters were played by beautiful and brilliantly talented Vivien Leigh.) Blanche DuBois admits that she has "always relied on the kindness of strangers." Although I am confident that the friends who have smoothed my path since my terminal diagnosis will stick around to the hopefully-not-so-bitter-end, I realize that I likely also will increasingly need to rely on medical personnel and possibly hospice carers, as well as people to help me with the mundane chores of life. Nevertheless, Scarlett O'Hara's famous last words also frame my outlook as someone living with a terminal illness: "After all, tomorrow is another day." This philosophy may seem more Pollyanna than practical, but it helps me move forward. What I'm not able to accomplish today I may be able to do tomorrow (although I recognize the danger of planning too many tomorrows in advance). Whereas my focus on gratitude is rooted in past achievements and experiences, I still have a future. Although the "journey of life" may seem a clichéd depiction of a human lifespan, I have more places to go and things to do.

I try to make my choices count. In 2014, roughly 12 million seniors lived alone, 32 percent of them women (American Psychological Association); perhaps my experiences and choices regarding dying or death may help other senior women, in particular, as they make choices about the life they leave behind and what is yet before them. Some days the reality that life is finite is more difficult to accept, in particular because I have had a "bonus" year of living as a "dead" woman. However, I must refuse to be seduced by this hiatus from debilitating illness.

Among the many wonderful days of December, the last day of a calendar year holds the greatest symbolic meaning for me. December 31 has always been a time of finishing what needs to be done before the year ends, whether that involves washing dishes or laundry or concluding reading (or writing) a book. (On a few New Year's Eves I have submitted a manuscript or proposal or nagged a co-author to finish a revision, no matter that the editor or publisher wouldn't read it until the following week/month/year; if a project was due by the end of the year, I took that deadline seriously.) Only after "chores" are done, as Dad said, can come play time. Whether I attend a party or count down the seconds to midnight alone, I always have celebrated what has occurred in the outgoing year, both the highlights and lowlights, and joyfully anticipated what may take place in the coming year (a graduation, a promotion, a publication). Every year, bad or good, deserves a commemoration and cheery send-off.

Some New Year's Eves were truly bad. During my teenage years, someone I admired committed suicide on the cusp of New Year's Eve. The worst was Mom's sudden death on our way back to Florida following a glorious Christmas at Bart and Nancy's Ohio home. December 31, 2007, was the day of Mom's funeral service, where I gave the eulogy; her burial; and the family gathering (with endless food and condolence hugs) at Aunt Bettye's and Uncle Hank's house. December 31, for me, is the ultimate metaphor for Death, and the Grim Reaper has often partied with me until Baby New Year is born.

On this year's December Death Watch, I walked Ormond Beach in the summer-like afternoon: clear blue skies, almost no surf, a breeze from the south, and chilly-but-not-toe-curling waves letting me enjoy an ankle-deep slosh along the sand. I picked up a black-and-white pair of cockle shells still stuck together after recently being opened and dislodging whatever had once lived inside. The shells' soft, dark moss-fur contrasted with the tiny sharp white shell ridges poking through. The exterior is all that remained of what had lived within, becoming the bivalve's physical legacy to the beach. The now-empty shells, connected by a still-tender seam of membrane, reminded me of both the transformation from the creature's life to death that occurred when the shell was fully opened and the metaphorical transition from being closed to being opened to something new took place. The shell was left behind for others to see (and, possibly like me, think about what was once inside). Someday soon my body will be nothing more than that open shell on the shore after I am transformed into something else. Pragmatically, that "something else" will be ashes to be scattered along the beach I walked today, with some buried next to the decomposed dust of my parents in the family plot. I hope, however, that my energy sent out over the years into the universe still will continue to influence others. Perhaps people will remember something positive I once did or said or will read or interpret something I have written or a photograph I posted.

Not all New Year's Eves have been so emotionally challenging. On every New Year's Eve of my childhood and teenaged years, my parents celebrated the new year with Bart and me. Close to midnight, Mom made orange punch with sherbet floating in the center of the fizzy goodness (a tradition that Nancy continues with her grandchildren). Our hors d'oeuvres varied by year and what was trendy at the time, from Cheese Whiz rosettes on Wheat Thins to finger sandwiches to Pizza Rolls to shrimp cocktail. With drink in hand, we stood in front of the television, counting down the final seconds until the Times Square ball fell into a new year. When Guy Lombardo or Dick Clark announced Happy New Year, we clinked glasses, sipped punch, carefully hugged each other during "Auld Lang Syne" (so as not to spill), then stepped outside into what, most years in Indiana or Ohio, was frigid air. We stood for a moment, looking up at the stars and listening for the cold quiet to be shattered by firecrackers or an ambitious neighbor's bottle rocket. Then we trooped inside, full of fresh air and a positive outlook, locked the door against the January cold and whatever imagined or real dangers lurked outside, and went to bed. It was a ritual, and I am a believer in rituals for their calming familiarity.

On what may be my finale to such New Year's Eve celebrations, my plans followed the time-honored ritual of special food and drink. This year more than one single-serve bottle of bubbly refilled my crystal champagne flute as I dined on brie. I stood to salute 2018 (and, in fact, my whole life) while I sang along to the televised Times Square renditions of "Auld Lang Syne" and John Lennon's "Imagine." Just past midnight, I heard Iz's "Somewhere Over the Rainbow/What a Wonderful World."

The pagan concept of the wheel is a powerful symbol that I embrace, especially at this time of year. There is a time and a season for everything, good or bad. (As the wheel portends, once I was the maiden, but now I am the crone. Sigh.) The seasons cycle around, and, as a lifelong resident of the Northern Hemisphere, my December 31 comes shortly after the longest night of the year. The end of December is a time of great darkness followed by the promise of the light's return, of death followed by rebirth, of an end evolving to another beginning. Within the wheel are many experiences that come in turn—some easy to enjoy, some difficult to endure. I can't stop the wheel, but I can acknowledge its inevitable turning.

I have had an incredible life, full of the joy of education and exploration of the arts, cultures, and places. I have met, learned from, learned about, and changed from conversations with the familiar and the famous. I have tasted success and been granted praise for my work as well as grown insecure from rejections and missed opportunities. I have done what I wanted and only regret the times I have inadvertently said something poorly or failed to show love more enthusiastically. I have been loved, as a daughter, sister, cousin, friend, mentee or mentor, aunt or auntie, lover or partner. I am joyous and grateful. If I had known my life was going to end this way, would I have wished not to have lived, or to have lived very differently? No.

Typical of my weird blend of secular and sacred texts as a foundation for my depiction of what comes after life and death, I find comfort in the words of my doctors—not my oncologists or surgeons but *Doctor Who*'s Ninth and Twelfth Doctors. Nine (Christopher Eccleston) reminds his companion Rose Tyler (Billie Piper), "Everything has its time, and everything dies" ("The End of the World"). A few years of television time later, Twelve (Peter Capaldi) adds to that certainty with this caveat: "Things end. That's all. Everything ends. And it's always sad. But everything begins again, too, and that's always happy" ("The Return of Doctor Mysterio"). As *Torchwood*'s Captain Jack, quoting T. S. Eliot, said, "The end is where we start from" ("Exit Wounds").

Ecclesiastes 3, Verses 1–8 provides the text first made hauntingly beautiful in a song by a pop group during the turbulent mid–1960s. Although the Byrds reworked the verses in their 1965 hit "Turn Turn Turn," the text comes from the Bible. The verses remind me to see balance within the big picture as my fortunes shift and to recognize the symbolism and reality of transformation and the ever-turning wheel. Hearing or reading the words is a comforting way to end this year in my life as a "dead" woman:

> To everything there is a season, and a time to every purpose under heaven; a time to be born, and a time to die; ... a time to weep, and a time to laugh; a time to mourn, and a time to dance; a time to embrace, and a time to refrain from embracing; ... a time to get, and a time to lose; a time to keep, and a time to cast away [BibleGateway].

This is the nature of life, as well as a fitting synopsis of the year since my terminal diagnosis. As the sun began to set on 2018, and on me, I still looked forward to the possibilities of a new day, a new year. I must live with cancer before I likely die as a result of it. Alexa, play "Turn Turn Turn" one more time.

Works Cited

American Psychological Association. "By the Numbers: Older Adults Living Alone." *Upfront,* vol. 47, no. 5, May 2016, www.apa.org/monitor/2016/05/numbers.aspx. Accessed 6 Jan. 2019.

Amit, Gilead. "How to Think About...Schrödinger's Cat." *New Scientist,* 27 June 2018, www.newscientist.com/article/mg23831840-700-how-to-think-about-schrodingers-cat/. Accessed 22 Mar. 2019.

Annie Hall. Directed by Woody Allen, performances by Woody Allen and Diane Keaton, United Artists, 1977.

Avengers: Infinity War. Directed by Anthony Russo and Joe Russo, performances by Robert Downey, Jr., Josh Brolin, and Benedict Cumberbatch, Walt Disney Studios Motion Pictures, 2018.

Blue Öyster Cult. "Don't Fear the Reaper." *Agents of Fortune,* Columbia Records, 1976.

Bohemian Rhapsody. Directed by Bryan Singer, performances by Rami Malek and Lucy Boynton, Twentieth Century Fox, 2018.

Boyd, Billy. "The Last Goodbye." *The Hobbit: The Battle of the Five Armies,* Universal, 2014.

Breeding, Brad. "Senior Living Pricing: Snapshot of Average Cost of Senior Living." Blog. *MyLifesite,* 16 Feb. 2016, www.mylifesite.net/blog/post/senior-living-pricing-snapshot-of-average-cost/. Accessed 1 Dec. 2018.

The Byrds. "Turn Turn Turn." *Turn! Turn! Turn!,* Columbia Records, 1965.

Carduff, E., Kendall, M., and S. A. Murray. "Living and Dying with Metastatic Bowel Cancer: Serial In-depth Interviews with Patients." *European Journal of Cancer Care,* 1 Feb. 2017, doi.org/10.1111/ecc.12653. Accessed 30 Mar. 2019.

Cargo. Directed by Ben Howling and Yolanda Ramke, performances by Martin Freeman and Simone Landers, Netflix, 2017.

"Catch a Falling Star—May 21, 1979." *Quantum Leap,* Episode 2.10, written by Paul Brown, directed by Donald P. Bellisario, NBC, 6 Dec. 1989.

A Christmas Story. Directed by Bob Clark, performances by Peter Billingsley, Melinda Dillon, and Darren McGavin, MGM, 1983.

CNA. Plus Academy. "How to Talk to Cancer and Dying Patients." *CNA,* cna.plus/talk-to-cancer-and-dying-patients/. Accessed 22 Feb. 2019.

Corpuz, Kristin. "Stevie Wonder's Biggest Billboard Hot 100 Hits." *Billboard,* 13 May 2017, www.billboard.com/articles/columns/chart-beat/7793055/stevie-wonders-biggest-billboard-hot-100-hits. Accessed 1 Apr. 2019.

Cosgrave, Bronwyn. *Made for Each Other: Fashion and the Academy Awards.* p. 112. Bloomsbury, 2008.

Daltry, Roger. *Thanks A Lot, Mr. Kibblewhite.* Henry Holt & Co., 2018.

Dickens, Charles. *Great Expectations.* Penguin Classics, rev. ed., 2002.

Dylan, Bob. "Knockin' on Heaven's Door." *Before the Flood,* Asylum Records, 1974.

"Ecclesiastes 3 (KJV) King James Version." *BibleGateway,* www.biblegateway.com/passage/?search=Ecclesiastes+3&version=KJV. Accessed 31 Dec. 2018.

Eliot, T. S. "Little Gidding." Columbia University, www.columbia.edu/itc/history/winter/w3206/edit/tseliotlittlegidding.html. Accessed 7 Nov. 2018.

"The End of the World." *Doctor Who,* Episode 1.2, written by Russell T. Davies, directed by Euros Lyn, BBC, 2 Apr. 2005.

"Exit Wounds." *Torchwood,* Episode 2.13, written by Chris Chibnall, directed by Ashley Way, BBC, 4 Apr. 2008.

Fantastic Beasts: The Crimes of Grindelwald. Directed by David Yates, performances by Eddie Redmayne, Jude Law, and Johnny Depp, Warner Bros., 2018.

The Favourite. Directed by Yorgos Lanthimos, performances by Olivia Colman, Rachel Weisz, and Emma Stone, Fox Searchlight Pictures, 2018.

Feltman, Rachel. "Schrödinger's Cat Just Got Even Weirder (and More Confusing)." *The Washington Post,* 27 May 2016, www.washingtonpost.com/news/speaking-of-science/wp/2016/05/27/schrodingers-cat-just-got-even-weirder-and-even-more-confusing/?noredirect=on&utm_term=.a873513d267f. Accessed 22 Mar. 2019.

First Knight. Directed by Jerry Zucker, performances by Sean Connery and Richard Gere, Columbia Pictures, 1995.

"The Five Stages of Grief." *Grief,* grief.com/the-five-stages-of-grief/. Accessed 21 Nov. 2018.

"Flashes Before Your Eyes." *LOST,* Episode 3.8, written by Damon Lindelof and Drew Goddard, directed by Jack Bender, ABC, 14 Feb. 2007.

Free Solo. Directed by Jimmy Chin and Elizabeth Chai Vasarhelyi, performances by Alex Honnold and Jimmy Chin, National Geographic Documentary Films, 2018.

French, Eric B., McCauley, Jeremy, Aragon, Maria, Bakx, Pieter, et al. "End-of-Life Medical Spending In Last Twelve Months of Life Is Lower Than Previously Reported." *Health Affairs,* vol. 36, no. 7, July 2017, doi.org/10.1377/hlthaff.2017.0174. Accessed 24 Jan. 2019.

Gold, Andrew. "Thank You for Being a Friend." *All This and Heaven Too,* Asylum, 1978.

Gone with the Wind. Directed by Victor Fleming, performances by Vivien Leigh and Clark Gable, MGM, 1939.

Gore, Lesley. "Sunshine, Lollipops, and Rainbows." *Lesley Gore Sings of Mixed-Up Hearts,* Mercury, 1966.

"Great News for the Dead: The Funeral Industry Is Being Disrupted." *The Economist,* 14 Apr. 2018. www.economist.com/leaders/2018/04/14/great-news-for-the-dead-the-funeral-industry-is-being-disrupted. Accessed 11 Nov. 2018.

The Hobbit: The Desolation of Smaug. Directed by Peter Jackson, performances by Martin Freeman, Ian McKellen, and Benedict Cumberbatch, MGM, 2013.

It's a Wonderful Life. Directed by Frank Capra, performances by James Stewart and Donna Reed, Liberty Films, 1946.

"Jane Goodall Responds to Ivanka Trump's Use of Her Quote in a New Book." *Inspired,* 3 May 2017, womenintheworld.com/2017/05/03/jane-goodall-responds-to-ivanka-trumps-use-of-her-quote-in-new-book/. Accessed 11 Apr. 2019.

John, Elton. "Candle in the Wind." *Goodbye Yellow Brick Road,* MCA Records, 1973.

Joseph, Jenny. "Warning." Scottish Poetry Library, 1992, www.scottishpoetrylibrary.org.uk/poem/warning/. Accessed 7 Dec. 2018.

The Judge. Directed by David Dobkin, performances by Robert Downey, Jr., and Robert Duvall, Warner Bros., 2014.

Kamakawiwoʻole, Israel. "Somewhere Over the Rainbow/What a Wonderful World." *Ka' Ano'i,* Discos Tropical, 1990.

Kansas. "Dust in the Wind." *Point of Know Return,* Kirshner Records, 1976.

LaPonsie, Maryalene. "The Costs of Entering Hospice Care." *U.S. News & World Report,* 1 Nov. 2018, money.usnews.com/money/personal-finance/family-finance/articles/2018–11–01/the-costs-of-entering-hospice-care. Accessed 22 Mar. 2019.

Last Holiday. Directed by Wayne Wang, performances by Queen Latifah, LL Cool J, Timothy Hutton, Paramount, 2006.

Leahy, Anna. *Tumor.* Bloomsbury Academic, 2017.

LibreTexts Project. Chemistry. "The 1st Law of Thermodynamics," 23 Jan. 2018, chem.libretexts.org/Textbook_Maps/Physical_and_Theoretical_Chemistry_Textbook_Maps/Supplemental_Modules_(Physical_and_Theoretical_Chemistry)/Thermodynamics/The_Four_Laws_of_Thermodynamics/First_Law_of_Thermodynamics. Accessed 7 Nov. 2018.

The Lord of the Rings: The Fellowship of the Ring. Directed by Peter Jackson, performances by Ian McKellen, Elijah Wood, and Viggo Mortensen, Newline Cinema, 2001.

The Lord of the Rings: The Return of the King. Directed by Peter Jackson, performances by Ian McKellen, Elijah Wood, and Viggo Mortensen, Newline Cinema, 2003.

LOST. Created by J.J. Abrams, Jeffrey Lieber, and Damon Lindelof. Bad Robot and ABC studios, 2004–2010.

Lovato, Demi. "The Gift of a Friend." *Here We Go Again,* Hollywood Records, 2009.

Love, Gilda. Directed by Lisa D'Apolito, performances by Gilda Rader and Gene Wilder, Magnolia Pictures, 2018.

Marcus, Greil. "Who Are You." *Rolling Stone,* 19 Oct. 1978, www.rollingstone.com/music/music-album-reviews/who-are-you-93272/. Accessed 18 Mar. 2019.

May, Kate Torgovnick. "Death is not the end: Fascinating funeral traditions from around the globe." *Ideas.TED,* 1 Oct. 2013, ideas.ted.com/11-fascinating-funeral-traditions-from-around-the-globe/. Accessed 28 Dec. 2018.

McLachlan, Sarah. "Angel." *Surfacing,* Arista, 1997.

Meah, Asad. "40 Inspirational Denis Waitley Quotes on Success." *Awaken the Greatness Within,* awakenthegreatnesswithin.com/40-inspirational-denis-waitley-quotes-on-success/. Accessed 11 Nov. 2018.

Midler, Bette. "(You Gotta Have) Friends." *The Divine Miss M,* AllMusic, 1972.

Mitchell, Bea. "Benedict Cumberbatch Just Ruled Out an 'Avengers 4' Comeback." *Esquire,* 6 Nov. 2018, www.esquiremag.ph/culture/arts-and-entertainment/avengers-4-doctor-strange-return-benedict-cumberbatch-ruled-out-a1907–20181106-src-esquireuk. Accessed 7 Nov. 2018.

The Monkees. "Last Train to Clarksville." *The Monkees,* Colgems, 1966.

Murkoff, Heidi, and Sharon Mazel. *What to Expect When You're Expecting,* 5th ed. Workman Publishing Company, 2016.

National Lampoon's Vacation. Directed by Harold Ramis, performances by Chevy Chase and Beverly D'Angelo, Warner Bros., 1983.

Nelson, Willie. "On the Road Again." *Honeysuckle Rose,* Columbia, 1980.

Oasis. "Wonderwall." *(What's the Story) Morning Glory?* Creation Records, 1995.

Ode to Joy. Directed by Jason Winer, performances by Martin Freeman and Morena Baccarin, Mosaic, 2018.

OncoLink Team. "Tumor Markers for Colorectal Cancer." OncoLink.org, 19 Sep. 2018, www.oncolink.org/cancers/gastrointestinal/colon-cancer/treatments/tumor-markers-for-colorectal-cancer. Accessed 30 Mar. 2019.

"One of a Kind: The Remarkable Life and Times of Senator John McCain." *CBS Sunday Morning,* 26 Aug. 2018, www.cbsnews.com/news/senator-john-mccain-his-remarkable-life-and-times/. Accessed 21 Nov. 2018.

Pantone. Announcing PANTONE 18–3838 Ultra Violet, PANTONE® Color of the Year

2018. www.pantone.com/color-intelligence/color-of-the-year/color-of-the-year-2018. Accessed 6 Dec. 2018.

Porter, Lynnette. "Love, Gilda." Facebook post. 21 Sep. 2018, www.facebook.com/ lynnette.porter.7.

Queen. "Another One Bites the Dust." *The Game,* EMI Records, 1980.

_____. "Somebody to Love." *A Day at the Races,* EMI Records, 1976.

_____. "We Are the Champions." *News of the World,* EMI Records, 1977.

_____. "Who Wants to Live Forever?" *A Kind of Magic,* EMI Records, 1986.

"The Return of Doctor Mysterio." *Doctor Who,* written by Steven Moffat, directed by Ed Bazalgette, BBC, 25 Dec. 2016.

Ryan, Claudine. "Stephen Hawking's ALS and How He Outlived His Prognosis by Half a Century." *ABC News,* 14 Mar. 2018, www.abc.net.au/news/health/2018–03–14/stephen-hawking-als-how-he-outlived-his-prognosis-for-so-long/9548110. Accessed 3 Nov. 2018.

St. Benedict Parish. Facebook post. 13 Oct. 2015. www.facebook.com/372634162885840/ posts/ the-bosco-boys-are-brother-steve-demaio-and-brother-steve-eguino-who-are-feature/535081169974471/. Accessed 1 Apr. 2019.

"Seasons of Love." Rent: *Original Broadway Cast Recording,* Dreamworks, 1996.

"Seneca on the Shortness of Life." Lucius Annaeus Seneca. Trans. Gareth D. Williams. Internet Archive, archive.org/stream/SenecaOnTheShortnessOfLife/ Seneca+on+the+Shortness+of+Life_djvu.txt. Accessed 1 Feb. 2019.

"A Show of Unity." *Victoria,* written by Guy Andrews, directed by Chloe Thomas, BBC, PBS, 10 Feb. 2019.

Smith, Kate. "All About the Color PURPLE." *Sensational Color,* www.sensationalcolor. com/color-meaning/color-meaning-symbolism-psychology/all-about-the-color-purple-4329#.XArPnOJ7k2w. Accessed 7 Dec. 2018.

Soylent Green. Directed by Richard Fleischer, performances by Charlton Heston and Edward G. Robinson, MGM, 1973.

Spider-Man. Directed by Sam Raimi, performances by Tobey Maguire and Kirsten Dunst, Columbia Pictures, 2002.

Star Trek II: The Wrath of Khan. Directed by Nicholas Meyer, performances by William Shatner and Leonard Nimoy, Paramount, 1982.

A Streetcar Named Desire. Directed by Elia Kazan, performances by Vivien Leigh and Marlon Brando, Warner Brothers, 1951.

Terms of Endearment. Directed by James L. Brooks, performances by Shirley MacLaine and Debra Winger, Paramount, 1983.

Third Star. Directed by Hattie Dalton, performances by Benedict Cumberbatch and Tom Burke, Western Edge Pictures, 2010.

"30 Pieces of Wisdom from Doctor Who." *ShortList,* 6 May 2013, www.shortlist.com/ entertainment/tv/30-pieces-of-wisdom-from-doctor-who/68791. Accessed 27 Mar. 2019.

Three Billboards Outside Ebbing, Missouri. Directed by Martin McDonagh, performances by Frances McDormand and Woody Harrelson, Fox Searchlight Pictures, 2017.

Tolkien, J. R. R. *The Lord of the Rings: The Fellowship of the Ring.* Mariner Books, reissue edition, 2012.

Villeneuve, P. James, and R. Sudhir Sundaresan. "Surgical Management of Colorectal Lung Metastasis." *Clinics in Colon and Rectal Surgery,* vol. 22, iss. 4, pp. 233–241, Nov. 2009, www.ncbi.nlm.nih.gov/pmc/articles/PMC2796099/. Accessed through the US National Library of Medicine, National Institutes of Health, 30 Mar. 2019.

Vitelli, Romeo. "Media Exposure and the 'Perfect Body.'" *Psychology Today,* 18 Nov. 2013, www.psychologytoday.com/us/blog/media-spotlight/201311/media-exposure-and-the-perfect-body. Accessed 23 Mar. 2019.

Weekend at Bernie's. Directed by Ted Kotcheff, performances by Andrew McCarthy and Jonathan Silverman, Twentieth Century Fox, 1989.

"Weekend at Bernie's Plot Synopsis." *Fandango,* www.fandango.com/weekend-at-bernies-126796/plot-summary. Accessed 22 Mar. 2019.

Wein, Len. *BrainyQuotes,* www.brainyquote.com/authors/len_wein. Accessed 6 Jan. 2019.

"What Does a Nursing Home Cost?" *Retirement Living,* 17 Jan. 2019, www.retirementliving. com/what-does-a-nursing-home-cost. Accessed 22 Mar. 2019.

The Who. "Who Are You." *Who Are You,* Polydor Records (MCA Records in the U.S.), 1978.

"Who Lives, Who Dies, Who Tells Your Story." Original Broadway Cast of *Hamilton,* Atlantic Records, 2015.

Williams, Pharrell. "Happy." *Girl,* Columbia Records and I Am Other, 2014.

Wonder, Stevie. "Superstition." *Talking Book,* Tamla, 1972.

Index